M000290980

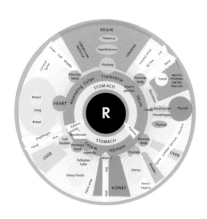

Practical
IRIDOLOGY

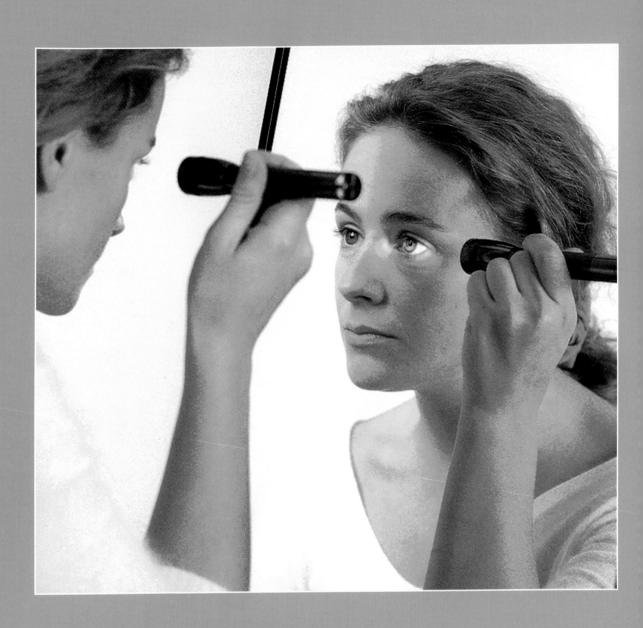

Practical
IRIDOLOGY

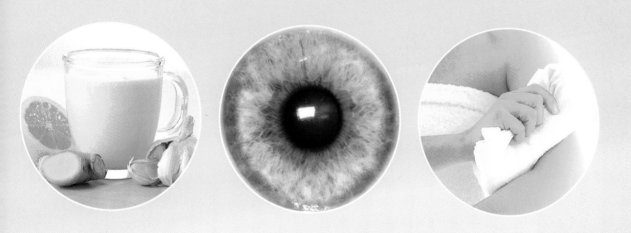

PETER JACKSON-MAIN

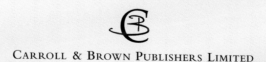

CARROLL & BROWN PUBLISHERS LIMITED

First published in the UK in 2004 by
CARROLL & BROWN PUBLISHERS LIMITED
20 Lonsdale Road, Queen's Park, London
NW6 6RD

Managing Editor Michelle Bernard
Managing Art Editor Anne Fisher

Text copyright © 2004 Peter Jackson-Main
Illustrations and compilation copyright © 2004 Carroll & Brown Limited

The moral right of Peter Jackson-Main to be identified as the author of this
work has been asserted.

A CIP catalogue record for this book is available from the British Library.

ISBN 978-1-903258-74-3

10 9 8 7 6 5 4 3

All rights reserved. No part of this publication may be reproduced in any
material form (including photocopying or storing it in any medium by
electronic means and whether or not transiently or incidentally to some
other use of this publication) without the written permission of the
copyright owner, except in accordance with the provisions of the
Copyright, Designs and Patents Act of 1988 or under the terms of a licence
issued by the Copyright Licensing Agency, 90 Tottenham Court Road,
London W1P 9HE. Applications for the copyright owner's permission to
reproduce any part of this publication should be addressed to the publisher.

The information in this book reflects, to the best of the author's
knowledge, current thinking on iridology. Neither the author nor the
publisher shall be liable or responsible for any loss, injury or damage
allegedly arising from any information or suggestion in this book.

Reproduced by Colourscan, Singapore
Printed by KHL Printing Co., Singapore

CONTENTS

FOREWORD

Iridology is the examination and analysis of the colored portion of the eye, the iris, in order to determine factors that may be important in the prevention and treatment of disease, as well as in the attainment of optimum health.

One of the advantages of iridology is that it can reveal many aspects of an individual's health. An iris picture may suggest that where there is a problem, more than one organ may be involved or that some emotional or mental element exists. This can lead to more appropriate advice being given with the person having a choice of treatments, such as seeing a chiropractor or a naturopath.

My training was in the School of Natural Healing—a school of herbal medicine based on the European herbal tradition and the native North American healing arts—founded by Dr. John Raymond Christopher. Dr. Christopher stopped at nothing in his efforts to heal sickness and promote health, and his reputation for achieving success in cases of almost hopeless severity is legendary to this day. His book, *The School of Natural Healing*, is a classic of herbal literature and a compendium of natural, non-invasive healing techniques.

The three basic principles of natural healing are simplicity, responsibility, and change. The simplest idea in healing is that you don't have to heal your body, or get doctors and specialists to do so. Your body heals itself, naturally and effortlessly; it is designed to repair and heal, and if it didn't, you would not survive. Natural healing is an affirmation of the body's power to heal itself. However, it also recognizes that for healing to happen, you must assume responsibility for yourself and make appropriate adjustments in your life.

There are many different methods and styles of medicine available today, but the only true healer is nature. The suggestions that you will find in this book are based on this premise. Therefore, instead of pills and supplements, you will find foods; instead of drugs, you will find herbs; and instead of sophisticated specialist techniques, you will find common sense suggestions that anyone can apply.

Iridology affirms the uniqueness of each individual, and the power of the individual to manage his or her own health. Your irides belong to you, and the information they hold is yours. Even if you consult a professional iridologist, you need to understand and resonate with the information you are given. It should have meaning for you, and be understandable in the context of your life. Knowledge, in this case, is the power to help and heal yourself.

Today there are physicians and healers of many traditions, and disciplines, including herbalists, homeopaths, and medical doctors, working with iridology. It is my hope that as you progress through this book, you will begin to share in the fascination of discovery through looking at your own eyes.

1

WHAT IS IRIDOLOGY?

Around the pupil of each of your eyes is a structure for which conventional science has as yet no full explanation. It is a recognized indicator of heredity, differentiated primarily by color: the iris (plural: irides, pronounced "eye-rid-ease").

The eyes and the skin surrounding them are indicators of a variety of personal factors. We can infer that someone's health and vitality is below par if his or her eyes are tired, bloodshot, or lackluster, or if there are dark circles underneath them; conversely, a sparkle in someone's eyes can show laughter, joy, or love.

From the earliest epoch of human civilization, the eyes have been used to impart information about their owners. The Chinese discerned health tendencies from the size, shape, and set of the eyes, and in the Indian Ayurvedic tradition, eye color is part of a person's dosha or constitution.

A PATHWAY TO GOOD HEALTH

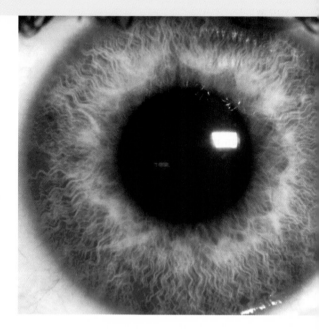

Your irides are unique to you. Among the five billion human inhabitants on Earth, not one has irides identical to yours. Not just the colors, but the myriad structural variations that can be viewed in each iris (and no two are the same) are the genetically determined evidence of your uniqueness.

It is estimated that some 200 differentiating signs may be charted in the average iris and iris identification is becoming more prevalent as a security device. Iris identification works by noting the distribution of distinguishable characteristics—striations, pits, filaments, rings, freckles, and darkened areas—within the eye's colored membrane and infrared light is used to reduce reflections and penetrate glasses and contact lenses. Your irides offer approximately ten times greater security of identification than your fingerprints.

A HOLISTIC PRACTICE
Iridologists believe that treatment and lifestyle strategies for individuals must be based on accurate assessments of the whole person and the factors that have shaped their lives. The "father of

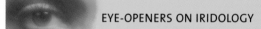

EYE-OPENERS ON IRIDOLOGY

In Greek mythology, Iris was the goddess of the rainbow who brought the messages of the gods to humanity. The full spectrum of the rainbow's color is symbolic of the diversity of humankind and reflects the great variety of shades that occur in this part of our collective anatomy: the iris.

medicine," Hippocrates, said, "It is more important to know what sort of person has a disease, than to know what sort of disease a person has."

Iridology, therefore, has at its heart the humanistic and holistic traditions of medicine and healing, in which the integrity of the whole person is observed and honored. It was, from its inception, a science that had more in common with the complementary practices of homeopathy and naturopathy than with mainstream medical practice, with which it has always had a somewhat uneasy coexistence. This is reflected in its history and in the experiences of some of its most celebrated protagonists, and continues to a large extent to this day.

Iridology depends only on examining the eyes; sophisticated scientific equipment or testing procedures are unnecessary. All that is needed is an ordinary magnifier, a flashlight, and sufficient knowledge to begin your interpretation.

One of the most common questions I am asked at the beginning of an iridology examination is

"Are you going to tell me what's wrong with me?" My answer is usually, "No. I'm just as likely to tell you what's right with you." Early in my career I developed the habit of ensuring that every first observation I made was positive. If you look into someone's eyes and reveal a catalog of diseases, you will probably frighten that person. It is much better to begin with some encouraging words to set the individual's mind at rest. Negativity will only reinforce an imbalance and will not promote a healing experience.

CONVENTIONAL DIAGNOSIS

At its simplest level, diagnosis means to determine the nature of a disease through examination of the indications. These indications include the symptoms reported by the individual as well as visible and hidden signs. A visible sign might be something about the person that gives you a clue, such as his or her posture, skin color, facial expression, tongue, pulse, odor, or vocal characteristics (hoarseness, for example). Hidden signs are usually the result of changes in blood chemistry, hormone levels, and internal tissues. Modern medicine has developed a range of tests from simple urine and blood analyses to surgical tissue sampling, endoscopy, and scanning procedures such as echocardiogram and ultrasound, CAT, and MRI scans to uncover these changes.

Complementary health practitioners are increasingly being taught differential diagnosis, which enables them to make the same initial assessments as medical doctors, through

logging symptoms, performing a physical examination, taking blood pressure, or palpating (examination through touch), and then determining which disease or condition fits the indications best.

These diagnosis methods are all disease-oriented, and probably conclude with the doctor/practitioner saying, "I think you have such-and-such a condition" and selecting a treatment to combat a specific disease. But how useful is this diagnosis to you? Does it empower you to tackle the problem? Occasionally, a diagnosis can result in fear and depression, as we struggle with the shock of hearing the seriousness of our condition.

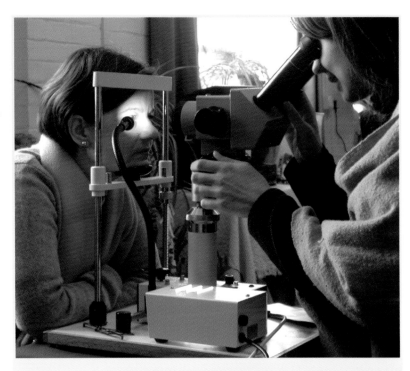

USING A BIOSCOPE When you have an iridology consultation, one of the procedures the iridologist will perform is to study your eyes and irides using a special camera. This creates slides of your eye, which can be projected and used to explain the practitioner's diagnostic process.

Prognosis

Alongside the diagnosis we also may be given a prognosis: What the likely development and outcome of the disease will be with or without treatment. In this we are entirely in the hands of the experts, and we usually have no choice but to believe what they tell us, which may not be what we want to hear. What power do we have to influence or change that prediction? A prognosis is only valid if you fit the usual profile of a disease-sufferer—someone who does not know how to maximize his or her potential for vibrant health and to take responsibility for turning things around. In fact, medical experience is peppered with stories of individuals who have disproved or outlived their prognosis through sheer determination and positive, creative energy.

> **THE PROGNOSIS EQUATION**
>
> **PROGNOSIS = DIAGNOSIS + INDIVIDUAL CONSTITUTION + CURRENT HEALTH STATUS + TREATMENT CHOSEN**
>
> **Change any of the above factors and the prognosis changes too. It will be obvious that constitution is a major factor in determining the outcome.**

CONSTITUTIONAL READ-OUTS

Some complementary health practitioners and doctors have realized that a disease-orientated process is not enough; lifestyle considerations, for example, have become increasingly important factors in determining health.

This is where iridology plays an important part; it gives you a read-out of your constitution, your essential makeup. Your constitution defines your health predispositions, not as predictions written in stone, but as guidelines to your body's innate mode of response. Iridology also may provide you with clues as to how your constitution has been affected by the choices and conditions of your life.

A blueprint for well being

This is more than diagnosis. If you know how you got sick, then you also know how to keep yourself well. What is important is the path that can take you back to wellness, and what you need to know to maintain it.

If you eat sensibly, exercise moderately, give up harmful habits such as smoking and excessive drinking, and manage your stress levels, you are statistically likely to live a longer and healthier life. When deciding how to improve your lifestyle, you need to know what is healthy for you, as different factors affect people in different ways. In order to do this, you need a method to assess your unique requirements, and this must be based both upon your current health status and your genetically inherited constitution. Iridology is such a method.

Iridology makes crucial information available to you—your strengths, weaknesses, opportunities, and threats. With this information you can make effective decisions about your health. It is just as vital that individuals assess their positive characteristics if they want to get well and stay well, as it is for them to be aware of their weaknesses and threats. The positive factors will be allies that can be relied upon along the way.

Positive factors may also tell us something about our path in life, what work we are most suited to, what we look for in our relationships, and how we seek satisfaction. All of these factors are vital in determining what changes we need to make in order to reverse ill health. People who exacerbate their weaknesses and ignore their strengths will not be healthy or happy. Also, what they perceive as weaknesses might be hidden strengths. Such weaknesses may be the safety valves that ensure any stresses we experience do not build up to insupportable levels.

Learning from symptoms

A symptom, usually a pain or an outbreak of some kind, is a message from your interior telling you that something needs to be corrected. If you wipe it out as an undesirable problem, using painkillers or suppressive medication, you are effectively silencing your own system and refusing to allow it to guide you. In this case you may be sure that sooner or later you will have to face the same symptoms or possibly worse. If, however, you listen to your symptoms and are aware of their significance, you can make the necessary adjustments. Even better, through a holistic health assessment method such as iridology, you may opt for a preventive strategy, whereby being aware of the potential for difficulties, you take preemptive evasive action. If you become aware of and respect your weaknesses, you can turn them into strengths, and thus also convert your threats to opportunities.

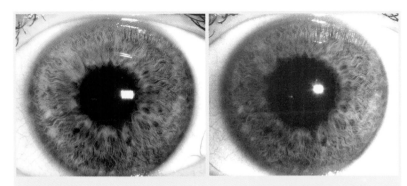

TOO MUCH MERCURY These are the irides of a woman who had been diagnosed with mercury poisoning. In the two years (approximately) that lapsed between the two photographs, the patient undertook intensive detoxification, working particularly on her liver. The "after" picture (right) shows a notable reduction in yellow pigment around the pupil and in the peripheral zones.

IRIDOLOGY TODAY

Iridology is one of a few disciplines that uses the eye in a diagnostic capacity. Ophthalmologists, for example, are able to identify a number of diseases by examination of the eye's interior. They also are aware of some of the signs recognized in iridology, particularly those relating to certain appearances in the cornea, which is one of the outer, transparent layers of the eye. Sclerology is another technique for evaluating health through signs that appear in the whites of the eyes. Like iridology, with which it is linked, it also is largely the province of complementary practitioners.

Iridology is now well established as a complementary health discipline in many countries. Due to its special characteristics, it has the potential to cross several boundaries specified by the modern insistence upon "evidence-based" science. From the detailed physiology of the medical model, through the approach of the naturopathic schools, to the broad-ranging skills of holistic practitioners, iridology has something to offer everyone who is interested in discovering the underlying dynamics of health and disease.

The study of the iris has also invaded the realm of the psyche. There are the beginnings of an energetic theory of health and disease linked to individual psychological and emotional experience, in which the iris is the focus of a holistic analysis of the multidimensional field of human awareness.

In the USA and Australia particularly, iridology has become associated with assessing the toxic loading of the body tissues and detoxification. In Europe, until recently, iridology was taught in some medical schools, and was informed by research conducted in medical contexts. The true picture of international iridology is that its different strands are now being woven into one. With excellent research centers on every continent, iridology may now be poised to break through the prejudices that have surrounded it, and take its place alongside more widely known medical disciplines.

PIONEERS OF IRIDOLOGY

It is not possible to say exactly where or when the practice of diagnosis through the eyes began. We suspect the ancient Egyptians knew something of iridology because in the Cairo museum is a display of painted ceramic eyeballs, complete with markings on the iris and sclera (whites of the eyes).

In the seventeenth and eighteenth centuries two texts appear: *Chiromatica Medica*, published in 1670 by Philippus Meyens, which makes reference to reflex sites in the iris and *De Oculo et Signo* ("The Eye and its Signs"), published in 1786 by Christian Haertels. But there was still no coherent theory or practice of iridology.

The story of modern iridology begins in the nineteenth century with a young Hungarian physician called Ignatz von Peczely.

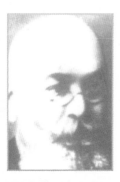

Ignatz von Peczely (Hungarian, 1826–1911)
When von Peczely was 11 years old, he tried to free an owl that was trapped in his garden, and in doing so the bird's leg was broken. As he nursed the owl back to health, he noticed a dark mark in a part of the bird's iris. Thinking that this was unusual, he continued to observe the phenomenon when the owl visited the garden, and was struck how, over the passage of time, the mark changed to a paler shade, as though it was a record of a past trauma now healed.

When von Peczely grew up he is said to have saved his mother's life with homeopathic remedies, as a result of which people began to seek his help as a physician. He began to study the eyes of his patients, making correlations between their illnesses and the markings he observed, and achieved great renown for his seemingly magical ability to read a person's health from the eyes. This soon attracted attention from the authorities, and an eminent physician accused him of fraudulent practice. Von Peczely responded by peering intently into the man's eyes and giving him an on-the-spot diagnosis, which was so accurate that the doctor withdrew his allegations.

Von Peczely was aware that there would inevitably be further skirmishes, so he resolved to train as a medical doctor. This enabled the initial development of iridology as a medical science, for it gave von Peczely the opportunity to study the eyes of live patients and of cadavers, and to link post mortem findings with iris markings. In this way, he was able to conduct a huge amount of research, which formed the basis of the body of knowledge we now possess, as well as providing us with the first attempt at an iris chart. Von Peczely published "Discoveries in the Realm of Nature and Art of Healing" in 1880.

In the latter years of his career, von Peczely struggled with the question: "Here is the sign, but where is the disease?" Signs in the iris were not always accompanied by ill health, and he struggled to understand why this was. In later times the understanding evolved that much of what is seen in the eyes is not the disease itself, but the predisposition to disease, and this forms the basis of modern iridology.

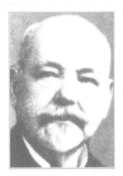

Nils Liljequist (Swedish, 1851–1936)

While Ignatz von Peczely developed his theory of iridology, Nils Liljequist was conducting research in Sweden. At age 14, the hitherto robust young man was vaccinated, after which his health deteriorated, and he suffered from frequent bouts of scrofula, influenza, malaria, and rheumatism, due to which he was extensively medicated.

At age 20 he published "Quinine and Iodine Change the Color of the Iris; I formerly had blue eyes, they are now of a greenish color with reddish spots in them." Liljequist's hypothesis that residual toxicity from drugs had caused changes in his irides was as important to the development of iridology as von Peczely's observations, and to this day there are iridologists who refer to certain markings in the irides as "drug spots."

Liljequist published his work, *Om Oegendiagnosen* ("Diagnosis from the Eye") in 1893. It contains a magnificent heritage of highly detailed drawings of irides, conducted before the introduction of close-up photography.

THE GERMANS AND AMERICANS

THE GERMAN TRADITION

Pastor Felke (1856–1926)
Felke promoted iridology in Europe.

Rudolph Schnabel (1882–1952)
Schnabel published "The Eye as a Mirror of Health." He discovered the iris sign, *Schnabel lacuna*.

Joseph Deck (1914–1990)
Deck founded the prolific iridology research institute in Ettlingen, Germany. Important work included his classification of the constitutional types based on color and structure of the iris. Deck regarded the iris primarily as an indicator of genotype, and held that iris appearances represented inherent predispositions. He published *The Principles of Iris Diagnosis* in 1965, which remains a cornerstone of iridology theory .

THE AMERICAN TRADITION

Henry Lahn (Dr. H. E. Lane) (circa early 20th century)
Lane introduced iridology to the US at the turn of the century. He was a medical doctor, and published "Iridology: the Diagnosis from the Eye" in 1904.

Dr. Henry Lindlahr (circa early 20th century)
A student of Lane, Lindlahr was also a medical doctor and osteopath. He published ``Nature Cure Philosophy and Practice" in 1913. Lindlahr's work emphasized natural medicine and the so-called "healing crisis." In the process of cleaning out accumulated toxins, the body may undergo a reactive crisis, whereby past illness and disease is partially re-experienced, and then released.

Dr. Bernard Jensen (1908–2002)
A pupil of Lindlahr, Jensen developed research on the "healing crisis." He studied chiropractic, osteopathy, herbalism, homeopathy, reflexology, and hydrotherapy and published "Iridology: the Science and Practice in the Healing Arts."

Dr. John R. Christopher (1909–1983)
A friend and colleague of Bernard Jensen, Christopher published "The School of Natural Healing," which forms the philosophical and practical basis for the Association of Master Herbalists in the UK. Dr. Christopher's reputation rests particularly upon his work with those suffering with supposedly incurable illnesses and conditions.

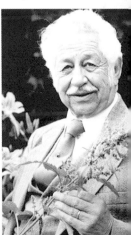

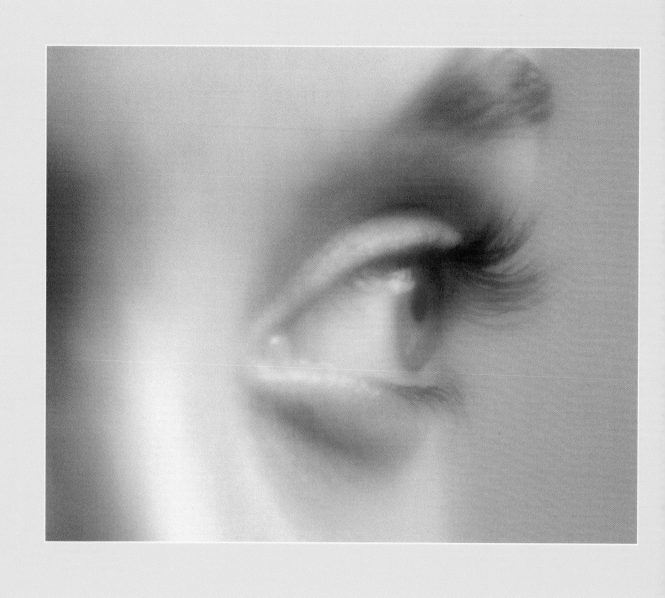

2

THE ANATOMY OF THE EYE & THE IRIS

By looking at the eye anatomically, we can uncover some of the underlying rationale for iridology. We also can get close to a scientific explanation for the phenomena that form the basis of the observations made by the iridology pioneers.

According to iridology, the function of the iris involves far more than the conventional medical definition: Operation of the muscles of dilation and contraction. Like the fingertips, the iris is very rich in nerve supply. The fingertips are highly specialized for the sensation of touch, yet the iris is not normally considered to be a sensory organ. However, experiments have been conducted in which thin beams of light are directed at specific sites in the iris, and the body's organs that correlate to these sites on the reflex chart have been shown to be stimulated. This suggests that light sensitivity is one of the properties of the iris.

THE STRUCTURE OF THE EYE

The eye is a hollow sphere made of a tough, fibrous material, the sclera, which is visible as the white of the eye. The chamber of the eye is filled with a transparent fluid known as vitreous jelly, through which light may be conducted easily without distortion. At the back it is joined with the optic nerve, a stalk of nerve fibers issuing from the brain. This is the wiring that carries the signals received by the eye back to the seat of consciousness.

The optic nerve enters the eyeball and then spreads around the interior surface of the eyeball to form the retina. It is upon the retina that the focused image of what we see is projected and then transferred through the optic nerve to the brain.

The tissues of the optic nerve and the retina are continuous, and this has importance for iridology.

The retina contains specialized cells called rods and cones, which are photosensitive, allowing light to be captured and transmitted along nerve fibers. Human retinal cells are then further specialized in order to be able to register light of different wavelengths—color.

Opposite the junction with the optic nerve is an opening in the sphere of the eyeball. This is the aperture through which the images of light enter to register upon the retina. Anchored to the edges of this opening are two structures vital to sight: the lens and the iris.

The lens is a convex slither of transparent tissue delicately suspended behind the opening through

A camera-like structure

The sensory cells of the eye are an extension of the brain, budding out from the brain during fetal development. Like a camera, the delicately suspended lens focuses the image on the retina, which contain photosensitive cells.

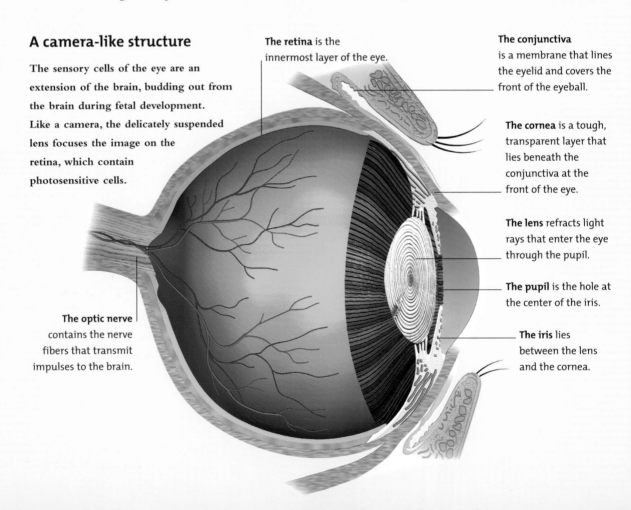

The retina is the innermost layer of the eye.

The conjunctiva is a membrane that lines the eyelid and covers the front of the eyeball.

The cornea is a tough, transparent layer that lies beneath the conjunctiva at the front of the eye.

The lens refracts light rays that enter the eye through the pupil.

The pupil is the hole at the center of the iris.

The iris lies between the lens and the cornea.

The optic nerve contains the nerve fibers that transmit impulses to the brain.

which all light entering the eye must pass, and which, like the lens of a camera, focuses the image on the "photographic plate" of the retina. Muscles attached to the eyeball enable the eye to focus. They alter the shape of the chamber of the eye, and therefore the focal length of the signal.

In front of the lens is the iris. The iris is a ring of connective tissue supplied with a musculature capable of contracting or expanding the space within the ring—the pupil—thereby regulating the amount of light that can enter the chamber.

Immediately around the pupil is the sphincter muscle. Like other sphincters in the body, it is a ring muscle, the operation of which causes the pupil to contract, limiting the amount of light that can enter. The pupil should contract visibly when you shine a bright light into the side of the eye.

In the outer portion of the iris are radial muscle fibers, which work to expand the pupil by pulling the inner edges outward. Our pupils naturally expand in poor light or darkness so as to maximize the intake of light.

CHECKING YOUR PUPILS

You can check the expansion and contraction of your pupils by shining a pen-flashlight into the side of your eye, standing in front of a mirror.

1 Flash the light repeatedly into one of your eyes, making sure that you are shining the light from the side of your eye and not directly into your pupil, which may cause you some discomfort.

2 Observe the changes in the size of your pupil. It will contract as you shine the light into it.

3 You will notice, when shining the light steadily into your eye, that after a short interval your pupil will expand again as your eye becomes accustomed to the extra light. This expansion represents an automatic readjustment to internal impulses from the nervous system.

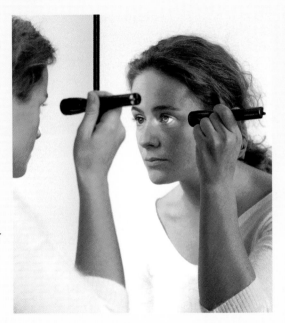

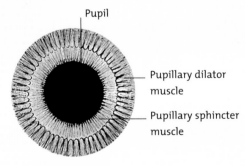

Pupil

Pupillary dilator muscle

Pupillary sphincter muscle

In dim light

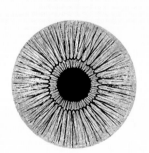

In bright light

Dilation and contraction

Sphincter and dilator muscle fibers cause the pupil to contract and expand, according to how much light is shining into the eye and the influence of the sympathetic or parasympathetic nervous systems.

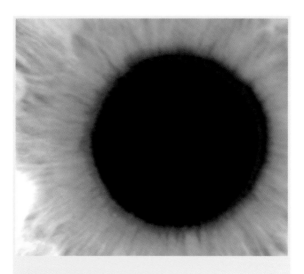

PUPILLARY RUFF

When the optic nerve enters the chamber of the eye it becomes the retina, and forms a layer over the inner surface of the iris. This layer curls around the inner surface, behind the iris, and emerges as a fine, reddish-brown ruff around the edge of the pupil: the inner pupil border, or the pupillary ruff. This structure is important in iridology.

Checking Your Pupillary Ruff

In order to see your pupillary ruff, you will need a pen-flashlight and a small magnifying glass. Or you may wish to purchase a "self-examination mirror".

1 Shine the light at your eye from the side, and look directly at your eye through the glass, or in the mirror, which should be held as close as necessary in order to maintain a sharp focus.

2 The pupillary ruff is visible at the border of the inner edge of your iris and pupil. It appears as an uneven reddish-brown ring, and it is normal for the thickness of the ruff to vary around the ring. This minute ring is the visible extension of nervous tissue, continuous with the retina and the optic nerve, and the only place in the body where such tissue becomes accessible to sight.

THE STRUCTURE OF THE IRIS

The iris is doughnut-shaped, and anchored to the shell of the eyeball at the limbus, or iris root, which is the visible outer edge of the iris. The muscles are contained in the deeper layers of the structure, but in front of these is the portion of the iris known as the stroma.

The Stroma

A body of connective tissue, the stroma contains thousands of vascular filaments and nerve endings. The filaments consist of radial blood vessels arranged in degrees of density, which vary greatly from one person to another, and also can vary within the different sectors of each individual iris. It is the arrangement of these filaments, or iris fibers, which constitutes the "iris print." Each iris print is unique and is used by iridologists to assess inherent health and personality trends. The density of the layers of fiber is a factor in the assessment of constitutional strength, stamina, and resistance.

The stroma of each iris contains approximately 28,000 "blind" nerve endings. These nerves can be traced back to an area within the thalamus known as the lateral genicular body. It is possible that here there are connections to all the organs and systems throughout the body.

Medical science has not yet offered an explanation for this phenomenon. One theory suggests that this circuit could form the basis of an internal feedback system.

Vascularization

There are about four layers of vascular fibers in the body of the iris, and these sometimes can be seen clearly where there is an interruption in the density of the fiber structure. A hole in the texture, known as a lacuna, allows you to see beneath the surface into the inner recesses of the iris. Sometimes a lacuna that penetrates the first or second layer of fibers contains smaller holes that go to deeper levels.

Occasionally, when an individual is under stress or feeling irritated, one of the vascular fibers or vessels may become engorged with blood and its outer sheath splits away to reveal a thin pink thread. While such signs are usually microscopic and not generally visible to the naked eye, these changes are important iris signs, and may point to areas of physiological stress within the body.

This complex vascular structure is not fully developed at birth. If you look into the eyes of a newborn baby, you may notice that his or her eyes are dark pools without differentiating features. In the weeks after birth, you will see some cloudy appearances beginning to form, the ghost of an emerging pattern, until at between three and four months old, the iris structure becomes fully formed. Pigmentation, however, may continue to develop even up to the teenage years.

Pigmentation

At the base of the stroma lies a layer of tissue known as the base leaf. This layer is pigmented a dark blue, and is the cause of blue eyes. The fibers in blue eyes are actually whitish or pale gray, and the blue color is a reflection of the base leaf through the fiber structure. Some research has suggested that this layer is receptive to light, and that a hole in the stroma permits the penetration of light to stimulate reflex sites deep in the iris.

The stroma also contains pigment-secreting cells that are responsible for brown eyes. The pigmentation from these cells is so dense that the fibers that compose the iris may not be seen. It is thought that the function of this pigment, like pigmentation of the skin, is to protect against strong sunlight, and therefore displays an inherited adaptation to a hot climate. In blue eyes these cells appear to be largely dormant.

Cornea and conjunctiva

The stroma is contained in its outer aspect by a thin transparent sheath: the anterior border layer, and then by the cornea and the conjunctiva, which is the outermost layer of the eye.

The anterior border layer and the cornea are important to iridology, as within these layers deposits, such as from medication, register as iris signs and reveal information about a person's health. The cornea is the location of one of the most well-known health-indicating eye signs, the arcus senilis (see also pages 64–5), which is related to the possibility of high cholesterol or cardio-vascular disease.

Autonomic Nerve Wreath

If you look closely at your eyes, you will see that the iris is divided into two concentric portions. Around the pupil, about a third of the way out toward the edge of the iris, a roughly circular structure is usually evident, which seems to be raised a little from the level of the rest of the iris. This is the autonomic nerve wreath (ANW) or collarette. Anatomically, it is a vestige of the pupillary membrane, an embryonic structure that ruptures shortly before birth. Its appearance varies. It is invisible in some people, while in others it is prominent and may appear jagged or serrated. Occasionally, it may circle the pupil closely and tightly, while in others it may reach out almost to the edge of the iris. Sometimes it is marked by a distinctly different color, which may radiate out into the surrounding iris tissue.

The autonomic nerve wreath reveals information about the autonomic nervous system, but it also represents the boundary in the iris reflex chart between the digestive organs and the rest of the system. Iridologists observe its variations, undulations, and degree of prominence closely.

THE IRIS' NERVOUS SUPPLY

Two opposing muscle systems—the dilator and sphincter muscles—are housed in the iris and they control the size of the pupil. The dilator muscles of the iris are mainly influenced by the sympathetic nervous system. This branch of the nervous system is involved in the "fight or flight" response, triggered by the hormone adrenaline. When you are under stress or are suffering from anxiety or shock, your pupils will tend to dilate. This is a physiological response designed to maximize the amount of information available to you at times of threat or danger. Nature knows that in difficult circumstances the slightest detail could be crucial to the preservation of your life.

The nerve supply to the sphincter muscle comes from the parasympathetic nervous system. This branch of nervous activity is paramount during rest and relaxation. The main nerve in the parasympathetic system is the vagus nerve, which is largely responsible for the nerve supply to the gastrointestinal tract, and it is this part of the nervous system that needs to be dominant while your body is digesting food. This is why eating when you are stressed or upset is to be avoided; if you are under the control of the sympathetic nervous system, you will not digest your food well.

EYE-OPENERS ON IRIDOLOGY

Sympatheticotonia describes an individual who is always on the go, worrying, anxious, or over-performing. Many of us in these days of fast travel and high stress are developing this tendency, and suffering from the inability to rest sufficiently. Vagotonia describes someone who may display an inability to get motivated, an apathy that holds them back.

These two branches of the autonomic nervous system are designed to operate as counterbalances, so that the sympathetic nerves help us to respond appropriately to the demands of life, while the parasympathetic impulses ensure that, when the action is over, we are brought back to a calm and relaxed state. However, some people may find that they become fixated in one mode—usually the

ASSESSING THE SIZE OF YOUR PUPILS

Studying the size of your pupils can give you a good idea of how your nervous system operates.

1 Looking at your own eyes, try to estimate the relative size of your pupil in comparison to your eye.
2 Shine a pen-flashlight steadily into the side of your eye. Your pupil will contract. After a short interval, your pupil will expand again as your eye becomes accustomed to the extra light. Remember when shining the light into your eye to let it linger long enough for the eye's initial light-sensitive reaction to subside.
3 A normal proportion is for the radius of the pupil to be approximately one quarter of the radius of the iris.

These are general principles, and your pupil size also changes according to how you feel and what is happening in your life. You can monitor this over time in order to determine the normal size of your pupils.

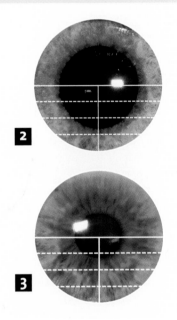

Influences on Autonomic Nerve Activity

Activator of Sympathetic Nerves
- Adrenaline, anxiety, fear, "fight or flight" situations, stress, exhilaration
- Drugs: ephedrine (used in bronchodilators), cocaine, LSD, cannabis and alcohol (first stage of intoxication), amphetamines ("speed" or "uppers")
- Withdrawal from opiates (reaction)

Effects upon Physiology
- Pupils dilate, blood vessels contract, blood pressure and heart rate increase

Activator of Parasympathetic Nerves
- Rest and relaxation, digestion, meditation, sleep, endorphin release after exercise
- Drugs: barbiturates, opiates, sleeping pills, benzodiazepines (e.g. Valium), "downers," second stage of cannabis and alcohol use
- Herbal remedies: "nervines" (nerve-relaxants)

Effects upon Physiology
- Pupils contract, blood pressure decreases, vessels dilate, heart rate slows

sympathetic nervous system. This is called sympatheticotonia, and describes the individual who is always anxious, or driven to perform constantly. On the other hand are vagotonic people, who may display a tendency toward sluggishness and an inability to become motivated.

Variation in pupil size also may occur with the use and abuse of certain drugs. Barbiturates, opiates, and other tranquilizers cause contraction of the pupils, while stimulating drugs such as cocaine, amphetamines, and hallucinogens like LSD characteristically result in wide-open pupils (see table, above).

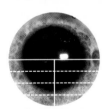

Extrovert
If your pupils are habitually larger than one quarter of the radius of your iris, you are mostly under the influence of your sympathetic nervous system. You will tend to be active, outgoing, open, and trusting, and to enjoy the challenges of life. If the enlargement is extreme, you may have a tendency to over-activity or over-stimulation of the adrenal glands. This can be a prelude to exhaustion, and you should assess your lifestyle and the demands you are making upon your body. You may be overworking or submerging your own interests in favor of others'. You may need to make firmer boundaries to contain and preserve your energy levels.

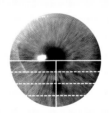

Introvert
If your pupils are generally smaller than average, you are mostly under the influence of your parasympathetic nervous system. You may be rather insular or introverted. You may not trust people easily and are careful how you use your energy. You are, therefore, not so prone to depletion and exhaustion as the "open" type. However, with the parasympathetic nerves dominant, there may be a tendency toward a lack of motivation, too much sleep, and lack of exercise. Think about ways in which you can redress this balance by becoming more physically engaged with the world.

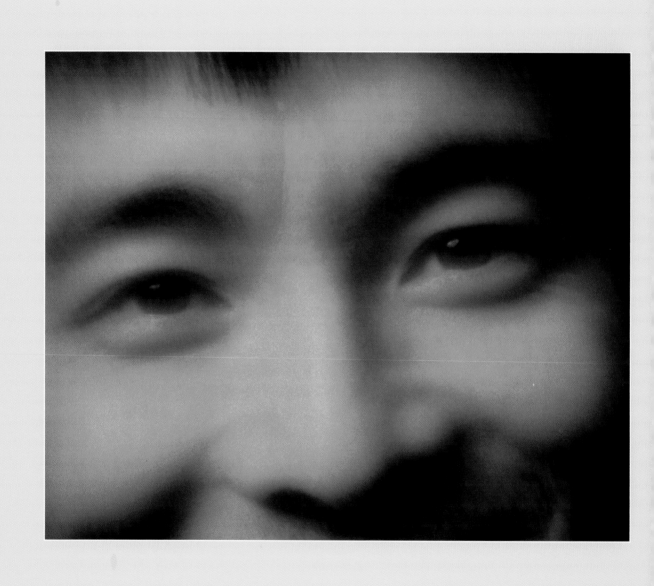

3

CONSTITUTION & DISPOSITION

Before you can look at an iris chart, find signs in your iris reflex zones, and link these to your organs and systems, you need an overview of your body and its susceptibilities. Constitution is defined as the sum of your inherited and acquired characteristics, and it depends on two main factors. The first is genetic material encoded in DNA, which governs such things as gender, height, skin, and eye color, and the second is acquired experiences in the uterus and throughout your life. How can we correctly understand and live with our constitution?

The three basic constitutional iris types consist of the two "pure" colors, blue and brown, and the mixed iris. These three broad categories represent different modes of human adaptation, and each one embodies its own unique wisdom and displays its own methods of attempting to bring an individual back to health. When considering the different types, bear in mind that we all are basically constructed in the same way. The differentiation in eye color places us in certain physiologically behavioral modes, but the same concerns of metabolic balance through nutrition, detoxification, and harmonious hormonal and nerve impulses are present in us all.

THE BLUE IRIS

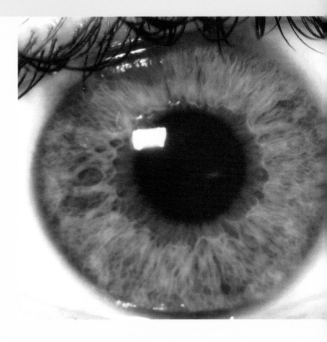

A blue or gray eye has no pigmentation except that reflecting from the dark blue layer of the stroma. If you look closely at a blue eye, it is hard to find any blue color.

The fibers of the blue iris appear as whitish or gray. If the fibers are not very dense, the spaces between them may appear darker and bluer, while dense, fine iris fibers will give a pale blue appearance, as they reflect more white light.

A LYMPHATIC CONSTITUTION

If your eyes are purely or largely blue, ask yourself if you have ever suffered from excessive mucus, frequent colds and sore throats, tonsillitis, glandular swellings, hay fever, eczema, cystitis, irritable bowel syndrome, fever, or rheumatic or arthritic pain. The key element in these complaints is reactivity. These conditions arise as a result of reactive inflammation in a tissue or organ. If something is irritating the tissues, the body will try to fight it. For example, when you catch a cold, the resulting inflammation is the body's attempt to fight the virus, which it experiences as an irritant.

"Lymphatic" refers to the system of the body that is concerned with the recycling of body fluids. By recycling fluids we keep the tissues of the body clean and unencumbered by waste products and toxins. Lymph, the fluid circulated in the lymphatic system, is clear plasma similar to blood, except that it only contains white blood cells, whose job is to scavenge for and remove debris, and to identify and kill anything that may be a threat to the system. In addition to drainage of the tissues, lymph is an active component of our immune system. This is why the predominant physiological concerns of the lymphatic constitutional type are elimination, detoxification, and immunity.

Derivation of Constitution

The blue-eyed type evolved in a cool climate (the northern hemisphere), where generating and conserving heat was a primary need. However, generating and conserving heat also leads to the increased generation and retention of waste products, which can cause irritation and inflammation. The volume and kind of foods—large amounts of fats and carbohydrates—blue-eyed types need to eat in order to generate warmth result in larger quantities of wastes being produced. Moreover, in order to preserve warmth, the skin and peripheral circulation need to be "closed down" against the cold. Normally the skin is an important organ of elimination through perspiration and "respiring" continuously—releasing uric acid, carbon dioxide, and other metabolic wastes. If the skin is closed down, it is less able to carry out these functions. It is also inhibited in other jobs such as shedding dead cells and collecting wastes for internal drainage in the "lymph zone" in the subcutaneous layers.

Blue-eyed people, therefore, have a greater need for their bodies to react so that irritants are brought to their attention. Reactivity is seen in the iris by the presence of whiteness. The degree of whiteness can vary considerably and indicates the degree of reactivity. You may notice that some stand out particularly, or may appear in clusters.

COMMON CONDITIONS

People with a lymphatic constitution have a tendency to focal infections and inflammations. Blue-eyed children suffer from runny noses, sore throats, ear problems, and tonsil problems. They also may fall prey to eczema, hay fever, and other allergic conditions. In my experience, childhood eczema is becoming extremely common among children with pale blue eyes. The condition is often traceable to an excess of dairy products in the diet (lactose intolerance is a medically recognized cause), together with a weakening of the liver, kidneys, and skin in their detoxifying functions.

Irritable Bowel Syndrome (IBS) is also more common to people with blue irides due to this type's tendency to greater reactivity. IBS is frequently connected with food intolerances and stress. What is often overlooked is that these tendencies are caused by the body attempting to find balance. Through inflammation and discharge the system reacts to, and tries to rid itself of, dangerous accumulations of pollutants and metabolic wastes.

Detoxification Not Suppression

Conventional medicine often tries to suppress appearances such as the reactions described above and fight the body's battles by administering powerful drugs— antibiotics to kill bacteria and steroids and antihistamines to suppress inflammation—or even

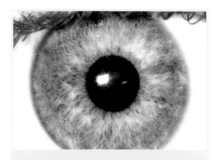

RHEUMATIC CONSTITUTION
The paler blue-eyed rheumatic eye is characterized by a general whiteness of all the iris fibers.

by cutting out an offending organ. The result of these strategies is that the body becomes unable to fight for itself, its immunity is weakened, and the toxic load continues to increase. The problems may disappear temporarily, only to return later as more serious, chronic complaints. A more effective approach is to attempt to reduce the toxic load on the system by promoting natural detoxification and eliminating harmful foods from your diet.

Unless specific steps are taken to completely eliminate toxins, everyone tends to accumulate residues of waste products. When this happens, your body may develop constant low-grade inflammation in its attempts to resolve the irritation caused by toxic substances. Over time, this irritation becomes destructive, leading to degeneration of body tissues and, in particular, diseases such as arthritis and rheumatism.

Blue-eyed lymphatic and rheumatic people (see below) are particularly prone to degenerative diseases. But by understanding the disease process, they also become empowered to prevent disease from occurring.

RHEUMATIC TYPE

A sub-group of pale blue-eyed individuals, the rheumatic type, tend toward exaggerated defensive reactions, though they are generally strong and don't fall ill often. If they get sick, they often have high, short-lived fevers and recover quickly. Their emotional reactions are similar: they may appear extreme at the time, but outbursts are infrequent and subside quickly. These people's irides are characterized by a general whiteness of all the iris fibers (signifying reactivity), creating a very pale blue eye.

Living with a Lymphatic Constitution

There are a number of factors within your control that can help you avoid the problems to which you are prone. Among the most important of these are the foods that you eat and the supplements you take and certain specific activities that will contribute to well-being.

DIETARY NEEDS

Water: Making up 70% of your body's composition, water is required for flushing and regenerating body fluids, and for elimination and detoxification. The "average" person needs about two quarts daily but you'll need more if you are above average in height and weight.

Fresh fruit and vegetables: These contain both high levels of water and of vitamins, minerals, antioxidants, and other micronutrients, which are essential for the maintenance of a healthy immune system. Fruit and vegetables, organic if possible, should constitute 60% of your diet, up to 80% in

Using hot and cold water alternately can stimulate circulation and move blood around your body.

warm weather. You may, however, need to avoid some citrus fruit (see Eye-openers box, page 28). If you have a strong digestive system, eat as much raw food as possible but if your digestion is somewhat "delicate," try gently steaming some vegetables, particularly in winter, to assist digestion.

Oils and fats: These are important for generating warmth, especially in winter. Linseed, hempseed, and olive are largely monounsaturated and contain a good selection of essential fatty acids (EFAs). Excellent blends of nutritional oils are available in health food shops.

TENDENCIES OF THE BLUE IRIS TYPE

- Naturally adapted to a cooler climate
- Prone to disturbances of the lymphatic system, the body's drainage network
- Irritability of the mucous membranes, especially the upper respiratory tract, but also the gastrointestinal and urinary tracts and the skin
- Raised acid levels, disturbances of kidney function
- Rheumatic and allergic reactions
- Easy onset of fever

Things to Avoid in Your Diet

Unfortunately, there are a large number of items that can interfere with the healthy maintenance of your system, including acid-producing and mucus-forming foods.

Dairy products: Milk, cheese, and cream are mucus forming and are frequently involved in disorders of the skin and mucous membranes such as phlegm, eczema, hay fever, IBS, and asthma.

Animal protein and fat: Meat, fish, and dairy products yield high levels of toxic by-products and can lead to constipation and consequent autointoxication, where toxins are retained in a sluggish or constipated bowel and leak into the surrounding tissues and bloodstream. Where elimination is below par, this is an appreciable health risk. Eat these foods very moderately if at all. If you eat meat, try to avoid red meat and pork and buy organic, if possible.

Sugar, refined carbohydrates such as white flour products, processed food, and food additives: These foods should be avoided as they upset the pH balance of your body. They break down in the system to form acid wastes such as uric acid and lactic acid, which are frequent causes of inflammation, especially rheumatic and arthritic.

Coffee, tea, alcohol, and carbonated or sugary drinks: These lead to increased dehydration and acidity and increase your need for water. Cut them out or reduce your intake.

HEALTH-PROMOTING ACTIVITIES

Skin brushing: Detoxification through the skin is a special need for lymphatic people, who frequently need to activate their skin. Perform dry skin brushing once daily, before bathing or showering. Take a fairly stiff bristle brush and work from the extremities in toward the heart in small vigorous

SUPPORTIVE EXERCISES

There are a number of things you can do to promote the movement of lymph throughout your body including yoga, t'ai chi, chi kung, swimming, and deep breathing. Deep breathing (see pages 118–19) is very effective because the main lymphatic vessel is the thoracic duct, which passes directly through the diaphragm. As the diaphragm moves with your breath, the thoracic duct is massaged, thus drawing lymph through the entire system.

The yoga postures in the Sun Salutation also are effective. Performing just one round is an excellent way to stimulate lymph. Other yoga

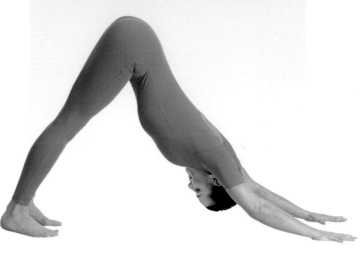

poses contract and stretch the muscles of the chest, arms, and shoulders, massaging the nearby lymph nodes and encouraging lymph flow through the area. Poses like Downward Dog work and stretch the chest, as do backbends.

Even a simple exercise such as bending backward over a bolster and stretching your arm over your head can be very effective at stimulating lymph flow.

CITRUS FRUITS Some nutritionists consider these to be acid-producing. Citrus fruits contain citric acid, which may exacerbate stomach acidity if you have a strongly acidic system. However this is usually because an imbalance is already present. Oranges are highly cooling, so are fine in a hot climate but should be avoided in cooler weather. Lemons have an alkalinizing effect on the body's fluids, and are frequently used in detoxification and cleansing programs.

BENEFICIAL HERBS

There are a number of herbs that you can use as teas or tinctures. See page 117 for instructions on how to prepare herbal teas.

"Alteratives" (cleansers): Dandelion, burdock, nettle, cleavers, yarrow, mullein, plantain, and red clover work effectively on the liver, kidneys, spleen, and lymphatic system.

Immune supporting: Take echinacea, elecampane, garlic, goldenseal, wild indigo, Siberian ginseng, elderflower, elderberry, and red clover.

Warming/energizing: Use ginger, cinnamon, black pepper, mustard, horseradish, astragalus, and Siberian ginseng.

circles, covering the entire area of the skin. Finish with large clockwise circles over the abdomen, following the direction of peristaltic flow of the colon. See pages 110–11 for more information on skin brushing.

Regular detoxification periods: Give up some unhealthy foods and drinks and drink more water. Cleanse certain key organs such as the liver and kidneys. Detoxify your system at least three times a year, especially when the seasons change. One week of detoxification three or four times a year can have long-term benefits for your health. See pages 114–15 for instructions on how to detoxify your liver and kidneys.

Hydrotherapy: Hot and cold water can be used to stimulate circulation and move blood (see page 112). Sauna and steam baths are also excellent, but don't forget to take the cold plunge between bouts in the hot room.

Echinacea has a reputation for minimizing allergies and boosting the immune system.

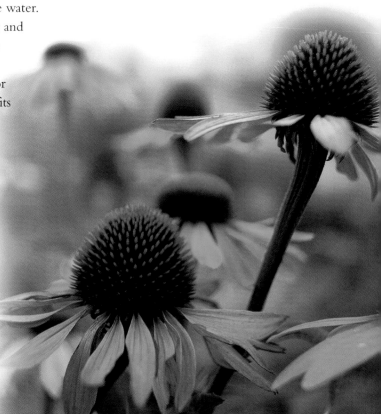

THE PURE BROWN IRIS

The color may vary from one individual to another, and there may be areas of darker or lighter pigmentation in the same iris, but generally people of this type are noted for irides that are smooth, homogenous, and of a velvety texture. The pure brown iris is sometimes described as a chromatophoric carpet; chromatophore is the name given to the cell that secretes this particular pigment.

The fibers in the pure dark brown iris may not be visible because they are suffused with thick pigmentation. This pigment is a uniform, velvet-brown, which penetrates all four layers of the stroma. Occasionally, it may appear that pigment is "leaking" from the iris into the whites of the eyes. Sometimes, in order to distinguish between the pure dark brown type iris and the lighter or more variegated types (see page 31), you will need to use magnification, as the naked eye will not pick up the more minute variations in color that reveal a mixed type iris.

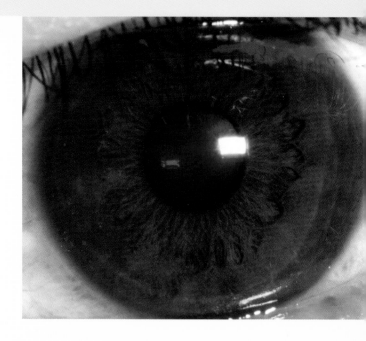

HEMATOGENIC CONSTITUTION

The pure, velvet-brown type iris is called the hematogenic type (from the Greek word for blood). The key indications for people of this type involve blood composition and blood dynamics: blood pressure and circulation.

This iris type's heavy pigmentation makes it difficult to see the precise arrangement of the fibers, and iridologists often complain that hematogenic irides are somewhat difficult to read. In fact, there is usually plenty to see, but this depends on putting in sufficient practice and time looking for the relevant signs and indications. You will need a bright light and good magnification to examine pure brown irides.

People with pure dark brown irides account for approximately 60% of the world's population so it is surprising that not more has been written about identifying their unique characteristics. While a range of subtypes has been recognized for blue eyes, and the various permutations and implications are well documented, only two or three subtypes are usually listed for the hematogenic type.

Derivation of Constitution

Pure brown eyes are predominant among African, Asian, and Oriental people. This fits with the theory that this iris type evolved in a hotter climate, the pigmentation being a protective measure. If you think you have pure brown eyes, check the color carefully. To the unpracticed eye, many very dark mixed iris types are indistinguishable from the pure brown iris.

There are some features in the iris that can help you determine whether you are, in fact, a dark mixed iris type. With a hematogenic type, the pigment is generally cloudy or patchy, and the depth of color may vary, and there can be light and dark areas within the same iris as well as structural features and variations.

Dark Mixed Iris: If any of the three descriptions below match your irides, you may have a darker version of the mixed iris type rather than pure brown.

- Irides are mainly brown, but there is an edge of green around the periphery.
- Irides look brown, but on closer inspection there is blue or green visible beneath the superficial layer, where it is interrupted by a lacuna (a hole in the texture).
- Irides are mainly brown, but the individual fibers are visible through occasionally thin, cloudy, brown pigment.

The Effects of Pigment

To understand the constitution of people of the pure brown iris type, we need to consider the effect of pigment in the iris. Pigment is thought to have evolved to protect against sunlight. However,

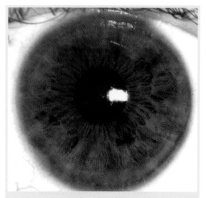

DARK MIXED IRIS It is often difficult to distinguish a dark mixed iris from a brown iris. The presence of blue or green pigment indicates a mixed iris.

the effect of pigment is to absorb light. The darker the pigment, the less light is going to be reflected back. We could say that the light "gets stuck" in the pigment. Pigment is therefore said to slow down energy, although it also could be said that it is able to store energy.

This may be another adaptive strategy, making brown-eyed people less reliant upon food for energy. Where sunlight is plentiful, less food is usually required. The hematogenic iris may act like a solar heater, absorbing and storing energy for later use. This stored energy remains in the iris where it exerts a continual influence upon the nerve endings, feeding sustaining energy back into the organs of the body.

COMMON CONDITIONS

Pure brown-eyed people generally have less reactivity in their systems. They do not suffer from the inflammatory responses or early onset of complications affecting the mucous membranes, skin, and lymphatic tissue that characterize the blue-eyed person. Brown-eye disorders are usually characterized by a slow onset and gradual unbalancing of normal function.

For hematogenic people, one danger is that problems build up unnoticed; there are not necessarily symptoms to act as warnings. Processes tend to be more hidden; reaction and inflammation are suppressed. That is why major diseases found in pure brown-eyed people tend to surface later in life and be relatively serious, being the long-term results of a gradual progression of metabolic disturbances. It is, therefore, important to catch and treat symptoms when they arise. For example, if a hematogenic person displays frequent lymphatic-

---

EYE-OPENERS ON IRIDOLOGY

LUMPS, CYSTS, AND TUMORS These are common among brown-eyed people. Tumors, thought by most to be a possibly life-threatening occurrence, represent an attempt to isolate toxic or potentially threatening material; hard deposits and formations are accumulations of matter that have not been resolved through normal channels and that must be kept out of the way of the body's normal processes.

type symptoms, which in a blue-eyed person might be considered normal, this suggests that the underlying disorder has progressed to a more serious level. Fever, for example, is a more serious problem for pure brown-eyed people.

Detoxification, therefore, is just as important to the hematogenic person as to the lymphatic. Accumulations build up undetected for years, and their influence may be more destructive for not having been dealt with sooner.

Blood-related disorders: Statistically, people with pure dark brown irides have an above-average tendency toward diabetes, high blood fats, and other rarer and more specific disturbances of blood composition. However, these are usually the full-blown end results of a lifetime spent in ignorance of this particular constitution and its needs. In contrast to people of the lymphatic type, where the usual need is to try and soothe or calm an inflammatory reaction—preferably without suppressing—people of the hematogenic type may need to stimulate blood, digestion, and energy in order to restore balance.

Blood tends to be thicker in people of the hematogenic type, and many brown-eyed people suffer from peripheral circulatory problems: capillaries contract in cold weather and the thicker blood cannot penetrate the narrow peripheral vessels. The result is cold hands and feet.

Stress and anxiety: The hematogenic person is particularly subject to anxiety and high levels of stored or unacknowledged stress.

Clots, stones, and lumps: The tendency toward accumulation and excess means hematogenic women may experience heavy menstruation, with dark clotted menses. Also common in both sexes are hard, crystalline deposits such as kidney stones and gallstones (often associated with high cholesterol), and lumps, cysts, and tumors.

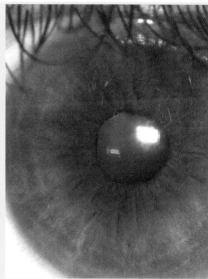

LIGHT HEMATOGENIC IRIS Look closely at this picture and you will see not only that some of the fiber structure is clearly visible, but also that small hints of blue/green are showing through in places. However, this would probably be classed a hematogenic type.

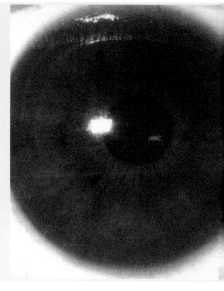

TYPICAL HEMATOGENIC IRIS There are variations in color even in the darkest pigmentation. Observe the very dark brown central ring, and the patches of lighter color in the main body of the iris.

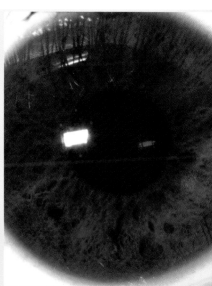

LOOSE-TEXTURED HEMATOGENIC IRIS Some fibers are visible in this iris, revealing a rather loose structure, with many lacunae and crypts. The mark seen at approximately 37 minutes is actually a dark "tar" pigment.

Living with a Hematogenic Constitution

There are a number of factors within your control that can help you avoid the problems to which people of your type are prone. Among the most important are what foods you eat and supplements you take, and certain specific activities that will contribute to well-being.

DIETARY NEEDS

Indigenous diet: If a hematogenic person is born in and has lived in a hot country and then moves to a colder country, he or she should adhere as closely as possible to the diet of the country of origin. Diets in hot countries often involve the use of peppery spices, which stimulate digestion and circulation. Adopting the indigenous dietary habits of a colder country, which include more fat, sugar, and carbohydrate, would aggravate hematogenic constitutional sensitivities.

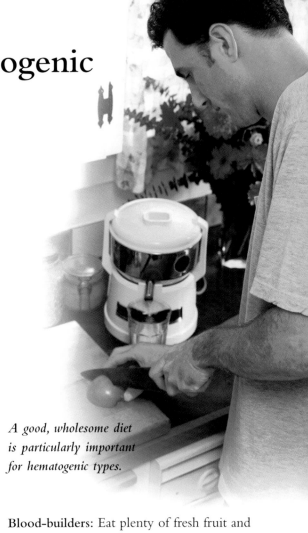

A good, wholesome diet is particularly important for hematogenic types.

TENDENCIES OF THE BROWN IRIS TYPE

- Naturally adapted to a warm or hot climate
- Disturbances of blood composition: thick blood, high blood fats, blood sugar abnormalities, mineral deficiencies
- Disturbances of hormone activity (hormones are transported by the blood)
- Tendency to excess and formation of stones and other accumulations
- Hidden or "sub-acute" disease processes
- Low reactivity, greater seriousness when fever does occur

Blood-builders: Eat plenty of fresh fruit and vegetables, particularly blood-building green vegetables and red fruit, for minerals and trace elements. Drink lots of fresh juices, which are excellent food supplementation. The nutrition in juices is instantly available and wholly absorbable as all the "packaging" cellulose is removed. The so-called "Superfoods" also can be used to similar effect (see page 123).

Things to avoid

Sugar: Especially refined sugar, to prevent or delay the onset of blood sugar disturbances and diabetes.

Saturated fats and cholesterol: Avoiding these helps to keep the blood unencumbered and reduces stress on the digestive system.

A HEALTHY LIFESTYLE

Moderate stress: Stress demands huge amounts of energy and nutritional power. The hematogenic constitution may not be aware of its adverse effects until they are serious. Learn to relax (see pages 118–21). Stress is a key factor in the onset of high cholesterol and blood pressure.

Keep warm: Try visiting a spa, keep active, and remember that your body needs to move. Enjoy its physicality and let it take you out of repetitive, anxiety-producing thought patterns.

BENEFICIAL HERBS

There are a number of herbs that you can use as teas and tinctures. See pages 116–17 for instructions on how to prepare the herbal drinks.

Blood-movers and circulatory stimulants: Use garlic, cayenne, and ginger for circulation and digestion. Garlic is especially good for high cholesterol, having the ability to raise HDL levels (High Density Lipoproteins). HDL is so-called "good cholesterol;" it transports cholesterol toward the liver for breaking down and eliminating. LDLs (Low Density Lipoproteins or "bad cholesterol") carry cholesterol out into the bloodstream, where it can build up to dangerous levels unless the ratio of HDL/LDL cholesterol is correct. Cayenne stimulates peripheral circulation, is heart-protective, and can help to clear deposits out of the arteries. Put half a teaspoon of powder in juice or ten drops of tincture in water or juice. Ginger is a circulatory stimulant. Put five to ten drops of tincture in water. All three have a stimulating effect on digestion. Black pepper, cardamom, cinnamon, clove, coriander,

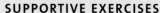

SUPPORTIVE EXERCISES

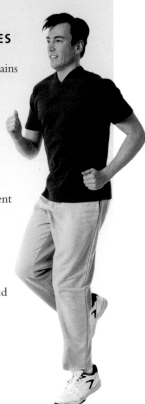

Cardiovascular exercise maintains the health of the heart and circulatory vessels, works against stagnation and cold, and keeps the metabolic rate from falling. Good examples are running, jumping, and swimming. The aerobic element of dancing helps strengthen circulation. Dance also introduces elements of grace and flow, helping to lift the spirits and keep both the mind and body flexible.

and cumin have an aromatic content and ease digestive sluggishness. Chinese Angelica (Dong Quai) is blood-moving, and can be taken either as a tea or a tincture.

Blood-builders (so-called "bone marrow tonics," or deep immune tonics): Use astragalus, yellow dock, Siberian ginseng, and Pau d'Arco tinctures, and reishi mushrooms, which are available dried or as capsules or tablets from health food stores.

Heart-supporting: Motherwort, hawthorn, lime flowers, and wild oat tinctures relax and calm, also reduce cholesterol and lower blood pressure.

Blood-thinners and cleansers: Take red clover tea, dandelion root decoction, burdock decoction, and nettle tea.

THE MIXED IRIS

Mixed irides, which include green or hazel eyes, may be very varied in the distribution and intensity of pigment. They may be quite dark, so that it is difficult to distinguish them from the pure dark brown iris type, or quite pale, as in the green iris type.

Generally, pigment is denser over the central region of the iris, around the pupil, and there may be some significant fading of this toward the edges of the iris so that the underlying blue or gray can be seen. The mixed iris type is also distinguishable by the visibility of at least some of the individual iris fibers, usually toward the edge where the pigment becomes thinner.

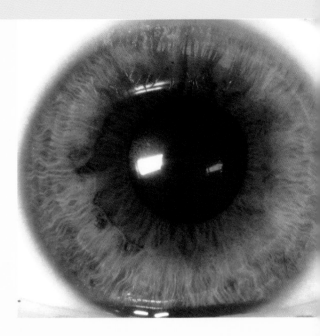

EYE-OPENERS ON IRIDOLOGY

GREEN EYES are not actually green. The basic color of the iris is either blue or gray, and over this appears either a thin layer of yellow or light brown pigment, or else specific, quite sharply defined, patches of color—usually yellow or brown. The eye of the observer puts this together and sees green.

DERIVATION OF CONSTITUTION

The mixed iris type represents two different sources of genetic information, and bears characteristics of both in varying degrees. Darker and denser pigmentation pushes the constitution toward the hematogenic iris type while greener irides may lean toward lymphatic concerns. Energetically, people of the mixed iris type embody a conflict between the slower, more measured process of the hematogenic person and the often intemperate reactivity of the lymphatic person. However, when the individual is in balance, the mixed iris type has the best of both worlds in terms of adaptation.

Whether someone is a dark mixed or hematogenic type may be insignificant, as the implications are very similar for both. In the same way, many blue irides have patches of yellow, orange, or brown, making them in between a light mixed type and lymphatic. Where pigment is a feature, it must enter the interpretation, and will inevitably modify the picture and recommendations for the types.

Digestive Concerns

Pigment in the mixed iris type is thicker over the central portion of the iris and this is where iridology charts place the reflex to the gastrointestinal tract, making the inherent health sensitivities of the mixed type specifically digestive.

The full name for this type is mixed biliary, a reference to the liver and gallbladder—the biliary system. The pancreas, too, is also involved, as it is a major organ supplying digestive juices.

The effect of pigment is to slow things down, and mixed type people have a particular tendency toward a sluggish digestion. There may be a reduced supply of digestive enzymes from the liver, gallbladder, and pancreas, resulting in discomfort, particularly when eating large, heavy meals or when trying to digest too many food types at once. Bloating, belching, and flatulence are common, and also a tendency to constipation.

There may also be *dysbiosis*, where the natural lining of friendly bacteria in the gut has become disturbed, partly through dietary factors, but also because of insufficient gastrointestinal immunity and an inability to prevent less friendly organisms from causing disruption. The best known example of this is *candidosis*, or infestation with the organism Candida albicans, which is also the cause of thrush.

Poor digestion may not always exhibit direct symptoms. The failure to break foods down and absorb them sufficiently can lead to metabolic deficiencies, for example of the endocrine system—the pituitary glands, thyroid glands, and adrenal glands; the pancreas; and the testes/ovaries. These types of concerns are also shared with hematogenic type people.

A CASE OF ...
Mixed Biliary Constitution

One person who came to see me was displaying many of the typical symptoms of a sluggish digestion: constipation, bloating, and discomfort after eating, together with belching and flatulence.

At times her discomfort was so extreme that she felt unable to eat, as every time she did so she became unbearably full and extremely uncomfortable. Her body was telling her that it was not a good idea to eat more food until her system had cleared itself.

The first task was to alleviate the congestion in her bowels, which moved typically once a week, and then with great difficulty. We gave her a lower bowel tonic, and once her bowels were moving again, her appetite began to return. We also gave her a bitter tonic to aid digestion and reduce bloating. The problem was almost completely cleared after only a week or two, although it was necessary to continue treatment for some months to prevent a recurrence.

URINARY TYPE
The lighter mixed coloration is often called the urinary type because the urinary system may be a particular concern of the greener types. People of this type share more of the lymphatic type's concerns about detoxification and elimination, due to a greater percentage of the underlying blue color showing through in the iris. There may be a tendency for sluggish conditions in the digestive tract to affect the kidneys, through the creation of toxins that slow down or impair kidney function.

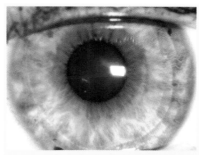

URINARY TYPE IRIS People with this iris type may suffer from sluggish digestion, which affects the kidneys, and benefit from detoxification programs.

Living with a Mixed Constitution

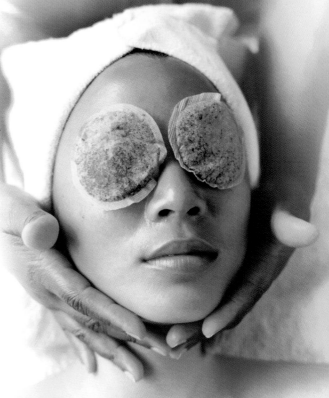

There are a number of factors within your control that can help you avoid the problems to which your iris type is prone. Among the most important are what foods you eat and supplements you take, and certain specific activities that will contribute to well-being. Make sure you also check the recommendations for the pure brown-eyed and blue-eyed types, which may be relevant to you.

DIETARY NEEDS

Food-combining: To avoid over-taxing your system, use food combining (see page 123). Smaller quantities of food, properly digested, supply better energy than larger quantities, which may cause clogging and fermentation.

Carbohydrates: Eat these in moderation so as not to overload the digestive system.

Juices: These relieve the load on digestive organs by supplying high-quality nutrition at low digestive cost, while assisting detoxification and immunity.

Massage is very effective for people of the mixed type, helping them feel comfortable in their bodies.

Things to avoid

Saturated fats: These are found, for example, in dairy products. They can be difficult to digest due to liver and gallbladder deficiency, and may cause bloating or nausea, especially if you have gallbladder problems.

A HEALTHY LIFESTYLE

Eat slowly: Take your time over meals, do not overeat, and concentrate on enjoying the food. Eating in a hurry places stress upon constitutional sensitivities and will result in disturbances.

Enjoy yourself: Pleasure and sensuality are key words for people of the mixed type, who have a need to become settled in the physical body, to accept it, and find peace with it. The parasympathetic nerves regulate digestion and these also are activated by recreation and relaxation.

TENDENCIES OF THE MIXED IRIS TYPE

- A blend of two distinct genetic sources
- Tendency to disorders of the digestive system
- Deficiency of digestive secretions from the liver, gallbladder, and pancreas
- Can display characteristics of either lymphatic or hematogenic people, depending on the degree of pigmentation

---

THE BITTERS In herbal medicine, digestion-stimulating herbs, including gentian root, century herb, and golden seal, are known as the bitters and are used to treat hormonal, or endocrine, disturbances. Without good digestion, the building blocks of hormonal activity are lacking so adequate mineral provision is very important to the hormonal system. Disturbed conditions in the digestive tract can sabotage this. Bitter herbs stimulate the flow of digestive juices from the liver and pancreas and throughout the digestive tract, starting in the mouth. Saliva is the second stage of digestion (the first being in the mind, at the smell, sight, or anticipation of food). Bitter herbs cool and drain the liver, increasing the flow of bile, and thereby also helping to relieve constipation (bile is a natural laxative).

SUPPORTIVE EXERCISES

After eating, walking or light recreational exercise is beneficial for digestion. Many yoga postures assist the digestive organs, for example, inverted postures (shoulderstand, headstand) aid bowel function and relieve constipation; twists and forward bends massage the internal organs; and "nauli" (the contraction and isolation of abdominal muscles) provides strong stimulation of the digestive organs.

BENEFICIAL HERBS

There are a number of herbs that you can use as teas or tinctures. See pages 116–17 for instructions on how to prepare the herbal teas and drinks.

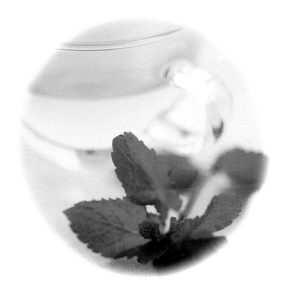

Digestive secretion improvers: Try experimenting with bitters, barberry, gentian root, century herb, wormwood, and citrus peel. Also, taking barberry, Pau d'Arco, walnut leaves or hulls, and Chinese wormwood will help to improve your gastrointestinal immunity.

Carminatives: Use peppermint, spearmint, rosemary, basil, and oregano to help relieve intestinal gas and spasm. Vervain, wild yam, and black cohosh work on the nerve supply to the digestive system.

Cathartics: Cascara, senna, and aloe will help move the bowels. Don't use these long-term, however, as you may become habituated.

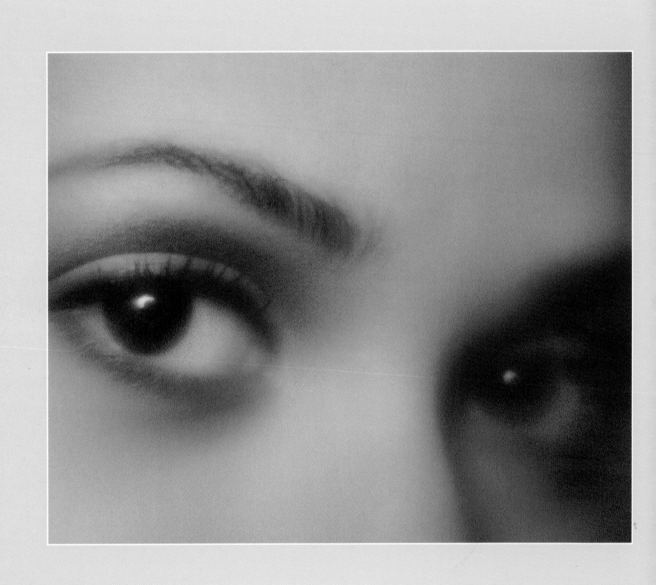

4

STRUCTURAL TYPES

The first thing you notice about someone's irides is their color. You do not generally notice their texture, because the features are usually extremely small. However, with good light, the irides' features can be seen even by the naked eye, and, with a small amount of magnification, they reveal the elements by which you can read a person's true individuality. In this chapter I will outline a classification system that differentiates between commonly seen structural types and their meanings in terms of physiological function and the energetic behavior of the body. This approach can be useful, but there are drawbacks. First, it does not include people who display composite features and, second, it relies too much on a valuation of strength without noting compensating factors. It assumes that a strong constitution is desirable, and a weak constitution automatically portends trouble.

It may not always be possible to assign a structural type to a person. Many people have a mixture of fine and loose areas of construction within their irides. In these cases, you should look at the individual indications as they are displayed, and, with the help of an iridology chart, make assessments concerning specific organs and pathways in the body.

THE HIGH-RESISTANCE IRIS

This type of iris indicates a so-called "strong constitution," and it is associated with higher-than-average levels of energy, stamina, and endurance. However, the keynote of people with irides of this type is resistance.

This iris type is characterized by a dense, closely arranged fiber structure. The fibers throughout the stroma are fine and packed together, containing few if any openings or lacunae. This iris structure is thought to be specific to the blue-eyed type. It is

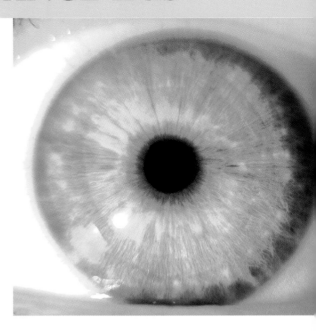

FIBER STRUCTURE

When discussing constitution, some iridologists refer only to structure and "iris density," describing a fine, closely arranged fiber structure as a "silk" constitution, which infers greater constitutional strength. The lower the grade of iris "fabric," the weaker the constitution and the greater the disposition to pathology or disease. The grades are described as: Silk, Silk-Linen, Linen, Linen-Hessian, and Hessian, or net.

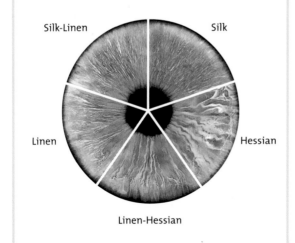

Silk-Linen

Silk

Linen

Hessian

Linen-Hessian

important to be able to see the fibers clearly in order to assess the texture. Density of the iris is regarded as a measure of the ability to resist threats presented by pathogens (bacteria, viruses, etc.) and other invading material. Therefore, these people often excel in fighting with their immune systems. Rheumatic type people, see page 25, frequently fall into this structural category.

But there is a need for caution. Because of higher levels of energy and stamina, there may be a tendency to overdo things and drive oneself too hard, and consequently these individuals are more susceptible to "crash and burn." I have seen more chronic fatigue syndrome in so-called strong iris types than in weaker ones.

CHARACTERISTIC TENDENCIES

"Strong" iris types are frequently found among care workers and those in a carer's role, for example the tireless mother who holds the family together and upon whom everyone relies. Equally, it describes the businessman or woman working late into the evening, seldom taking holidays, and relying too much on caffeine to power his or her adrenal glands.

Strong iris types tend to leave little time to relax, and have less opportunity to discharge accumulated stress. Because of this, they eventually hit the brick wall harder. Most people with this pattern need to learn to slow down, relax, take breaks, and find a way of dispersing the pressure.

Energetically, these people are kinesthetic types: good communicators, action-oriented, and practical. They can be very sensitive, and may tend to hold a lot inside and not process their emotions fully, so that these build up, adding to the pressure.

Their strong capacity for resistance has both positive and negative effects. As well as resisting damaging factors such as bacteria, they also can resist positive influences. It may be difficult to give them advice, because they know best and they sometimes cannot listen. Motivating a high resistance type person will depend on the use of practical demonstration and giving him or her hands-on experience.

If energy input is balanced with expenditure, people of this type can be the most efficient. However, they are susceptible to overextending, and, as a result, may suffer from disorders of the nervous system, minor cramps and ticks through neuroses and depression, and more serious pathologies such as multiple sclerosis and motor neurone disease, although these are rare.

There are two subtypes within this category.

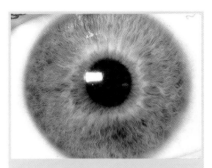

RESISTANCE-ROBUST IRIS
These people often find it difficult to relax unless they push themselves to the limit through extreme forms of exercise.

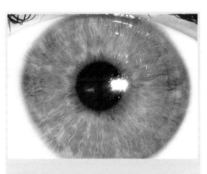

RESISTANCE-SENSITIVE IRIS
These people tend toward anxiety and are sensitive to harsh surroundings, including aggressive or intrusive people.

HIGH RESISTANCE-ROBUST TYPE

The term "adrenaline junkie" can describe this type. These people tend toward feats of physical endurance and daring, with little regard for safety. They find it hard to relax unless pushed to the limits and often choose extreme sports to unwind, using the endorphin release following the output of adrenaline.

These people have "silk" textured irides (see box left) with few—if any—holes or gaps in the texture. The surface layer of the iris stroma has a wavy appearance, often described as "combed hair," as it stretches out from the collarette to the edge of the iris. The collarette is prominent and bright white in color, indicating hyperactivity of the autonomic nerve system.

HIGH RESISTANCE-SENSITIVE TYPE

These people are strong, but have a tendency toward worry and anxiety. They have finely tuned nervous systems and are vulnerable to harsh or intrusive stimuli, including the negative emotions of people around them.

High resistance-sensitive types have very fine iris fibers, closely packed, and with a very fine "silk" texture. But the collarette in this type is much less prominent than in the high resistance-robust type, sometimes almost invisible. There may be circular features, which are contraction furrows—ripple-like grooves around the iris.

Living with a High-Resistance Constitution

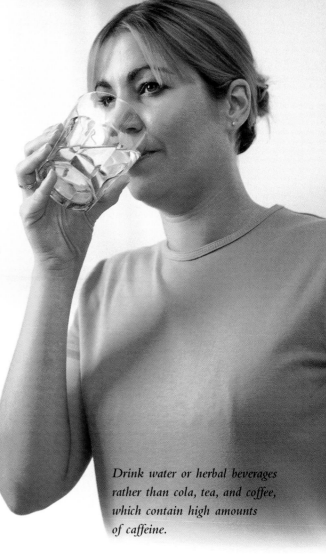

There are various recommendations for what to eat, how to exercise, and other lifestyle changes that should be followed. Combine these with those already given for blue-eyed people.

DIETARY NEEDS

Nerve-building foods and supplements: Oats and lecithin are effective.

Whole grains: A highly useful food class for high resistance people, always choose whole grains, such as oats, barley, buckwheat, and quinoa.

Things to avoid

Sugar and caffeine: Since you have a high energy consumption, carbohydrates are in big demand, but don't be tempted to compromise health by overindulging in refined carbohydrates and caffeine: these will lift energy levels for a short period but will not sustain them, and will have undesirable long-term consequences. It may be difficult to give these up and you will need to use strategies such as visualizations or meditation, stretching exercises, or deep breathing (see pages 118–122). Substituting water or a herbal drink for tea and coffee, and fruit and nuts to replace sugar and high-calorie snacks will help.

Drink water or herbal beverages rather than cola, tea, and coffee, which contain high amounts of caffeine.

HEALTHY LIFESTYLE

Relax: Pace yourself to ensure that you make the most of your above average strength and endurance. You are rarely still, either physically or mentally, so use exercise routines such as yoga or t'ai chi to help you relax.

Learn to say "No": You need to refuse to do things occasionally, to prevent yourself becoming over-committed. Even though you can accomplish most tasks faster than other people, you must learn to restrain yourself.

Look after yourself: Most high resistance type people (especially high resistance-robust types) are irritated by illness and don't have time for it. You tend to smother symptoms with painkillers and ignore them. You can do this for years and not notice the wear and tear, but you will pay for it later with more serious symptoms.

Love yourself: You are your own harshest critic and better at looking after others than yourself.

Make lifestyle changes: If healing is to be achieved, you must adhere to lifestyle changes. If you cause a relapse of an illness, it may be more difficult to recover in subsequent times. Illness needs to be addressed by reevaluating your lifestyle.

BENEFICIAL HERBS

There are a number of herbs that you can use as teas or tinctures. See pages 116–17 for instructions on how to prepare the herbal drinks.

Nerve-builders: Nervines nourish and relax the nervous system. Use wild oat, vervain, lime flowers, chamomile, skullcap, ashwagandha, hops, and passionflower. Valerian is an excellent source of calcium—a mineral used in large quantities by the nervous system.

Stress-busters and stamina-builders: Adaptogenics are also adrenal and bone marrow tonics. Use ginseng (any variety), wild oat, Pau d'Arco, astragalus, and licorice.

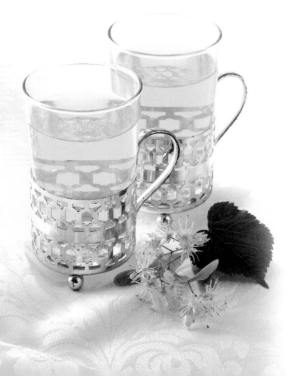

SUPPORTIVE EXERCISES

Because of your reserves of strength and stamina, you like demanding exercise, and you need to exert yourself occasionally. This is because your nervous activity tends to produce large quantities of the chemical acetylcholine at the nerve synapses. The synapse occurs at the gap between nerve cells. The nerve impulse is fired across the gap assisted by chemicals known as neurotransmitters, one of which is acetylcholine. Exercise is a very efficient way of using up excessive acetylcholine. A buildup of this chemical may result in restlessness or twitchiness.

Aerobic exercise is powered by the sympathetic nervous system, and there is an automatic synergistic reaction whereby after exercising, the parasympathetic nervous system assumes dominance through the release of the hormone endorphin, which is chemically similar to opiates. This "endorphin kick" calms, relaxes, and stills the body and mind. Activities such as meditation are easier for you after vigorous exercise.

THE CONNECTIVE TISSUE-RECEPTIVE IRIS

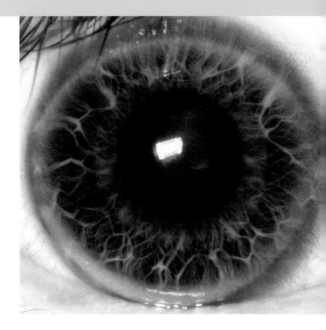

At the opposite extreme from the high-resistance type are people of the connective tissue-receptive type. The former type's close-textured iris is responsible for its emphasis upon resistance. The reverse is true of the connective tissue-receptive person. This individual does not resist well and is at a higher risk of attracting damaging pathological influences.

The connective tissue-receptive person, however, does have an adaptive sensitivity, which can be an advantage. These people are emotionally open and receptive in a positive way. And while this iris type is considered specific to people with blue eyes, the quality of greater openness can apply to all colors.

The connective tissue-receptive disposition is described as a low-density iris, where the fibers are much less numerous than in the high resistance iris type. The color is darker, with the exception of bright individual fibers. The stroma of the iris is therefore more penetrable than other types. This means that more light can enter the inner levels of the iris and stimulate reflex sites and nerve endings, which may be an advantageous adaptation strategy.

Traditionally, areas of open structure are regarded as indicative of weakness in the organs linked reflexively to the site and should be taken seriously as targets for treatment. This openness implies a less robust constitution than that of the high resistance iris type, and yet its sensitivity is considered its chief advantage.

CHARACTERISTIC TENDENCIES

Connective tissue-receptive people rely on energy conservation and prudence. Conscious of their limits, these people will pull back from over-stretching and retire to regenerate. Knowing that they do not heal as easily as others, they will not readily put themselves in dangerous situations. However, when pressured, these people's openness is an advantage. In difficult situations, keeping your ears and eyes open is a good strategy for survival.

Physiologically, these people tend to suffer from connective tissue disorders. There may be difficulty in transporting oxygen and nutrients to where they are needed, and drainage may be poor, resulting in retention of fluids (edema) and toxicity of tissues. This amplifies the key themes of lymphatic people. Deficiency of connective tissue also may result in the prolapse of organs.

Connective tissue-receptive people need to look after themselves and they are usually aware of this. Receptivity is key for these open people. They take advice seriously, and audio tapes and other programs for self-development, music, and chanting all can be used in healing.

Living with a Connective Tissue-Receptive Constitution

The true connective tissue-receptive iris is relatively rare, and there are degrees of openness within people of this type. It is perfectly possible for these people to live in harmony with their constitution. This constitution is found most often in lymphatic people, where there is an increased tendency to retain due to slower than average drainage. Therefore, you also should refer to suggestions for the lymphatic iris type.

DIETARY NEEDS

Fresh produce: Eat plenty of fruit and vegetables rich in essential nutrients such as vitamins, especially those high in vitamin C, minerals, trace elements, and antioxidants. Oranges, blackcurrants, strawberries, potatoes, Brussels sprouts, broccoli, green leafy vegetables, green peppers and parsley are all good choices.

Detoxification: Eat foods that gently assist elimination and do not add to toxic residues, such as fresh fruit (high in vitamin C, antioxidants, and water content). In addition to the fruit and vegetables listed above, all red fruits (such as blackberries, raspberries, redcurrants, bilberries, and cranberries), and fruit and vegetable juices are ideal. Juicing maximizes the mineral and vitamin absorption from the foods juiced. Also, certain "superfoods" such as spirulina, chlorella, and alfalfa are beneficial (see page 123).

A HEALTHY LIFESTYLE

Relax and regenerate: Connective tissue-receptive individuals have less stamina than others and should not be pushed too hard. If this is your type, make sure you allow sufficient time for relaxation

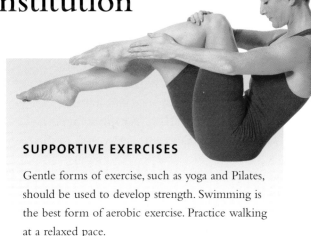

SUPPORTIVE EXERCISES

Gentle forms of exercise, such as yoga and Pilates, should be used to develop strength. Swimming is the best form of aerobic exercise. Practice walking at a relaxed pace.

and regeneration. Take care that your lifestyle does not demand too much of you. Learn to measure your pace and find ways to relax.

Avoid strenuous exercise: Connective tissue sensitivity makes it unwise to engage in demanding exercise and you are very susceptible to cartilage and joint problems, internal organ displacement, and the early onset of arthritis.

BENEFICIAL HERBS

A number of herbs can be used as teas or tinctures. See page 116 for how to prepare herbal drinks.

Immunity stimulants and protectors: Use echinacea, elder, elecampane, eucalyptus, garlic, schisandra, wild indigo, and wild cherry.

Stamina-building: Take astragalus, Siberian ginseng, borage, wild oat, and gotu kola.

Detoxifying: Detoxify slowly, using diet as the foundation. Use local herbs such as dandelion, nettle, cleavers, dock, and burdock.

THE SELF-PROTECTIVE IRIS

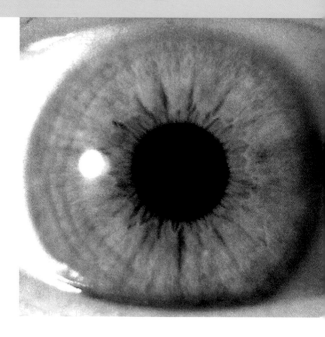

Self-protective people are related to high-resistance individuals, both having dense irides. They construct highly effective defenses, often physical, which allow them to focus and screen out unwanted impressions.

Like individuals of the high-resistance type, these people are kinesthetic and "doers." They may be found at the top of their professions, exhibiting calm, rational behavior that inspires confidence. The characteristic iris features of self-protective people include contraction furrows—at least three or four concentric circular grooves in the iris—and radial furrows. The latter can be major—deep troughs that radiate outward from the pupil margin, cutting through the collarette, into the ciliary zone, or minor—smaller and less deep, which start at the collarette.

CHARACTERISTIC TENDENCIES

Self-protective people, like high resistance-individuals, may be driven by anxiety. The defenses also represent fear, leading to a need for withdrawal. A confident exterior frequently masks a vulnerable inner world, and the protective patterns shield them from a harsh environment.

These people are socially aware and effective: the radial furrows, like sun rays, represent openness. A strategy of withdrawal helps them to perform with confidence, keeping people unaware of their sensitivity. On one hand there is openness; on the other there is retreat. These people always go back to their own space for regrouping.

Physiologically, self-protective individuals also resemble high-resistance people. However, the maintenance of muscular contractions—a part of their defensive reactions—demands large amounts of energy. There is increased pressure on gastrointestinal dynamics to supply this energy. This, combined with the presence of radial furrows, which cut through the collarette, and indicate that the nerve supply to the digestive organs may be affected, points to the potential for a damaging "energy gap" to appear, especially under stress. These people often feel very tired and may suffer from tension and pain but they respond well to massage therapies. Cramps (including menstrual cramps, for women), tics, spasms, and muscular tension are also common.

These iris types are most frequently found among the hematogenic and mixed iris types, which emphasize the need to care for gastrointestinal health. However, the pattern is increasingly found in lymphatic people, as an intensification of the high resistance-sensitive type. Whichever color type you are, the health of your digestive organs is crucial to your ability to perform, and excellent nutrition is essential.

Living with a Self-Protective Constitution

There are several factors that can help you avoid the problems to which you are prone, including the foods you eat and performing exercises that assist the functioning of the digestive system. Make sure also to check the recommendations for your relevant color type.

DIETARY NEEDS

Juices and "superfoods": These will ensure that you receive a high mineral intake and uptake (see page 123 for information on superfoods).

Nerve builders: You need to eat foods that nourish your nervous system. Such foods are high in B vitamins, and include whole grains, nutritional yeast, wheatgerm, beansprouts, avocados, nuts, mushrooms, and green leafy vegetables. You also need to take more calcium, which is found in green vegetables, oranges, almonds, and tofu; and the co-factors essential for the absorption of calcium, such as vitamins A and C, found in citrus fruit and berries, and magnesium, found in nuts, bananas, and soya beans.

A HEALTHY LIFESTYLE

Balance: Measured rest and work ratios are essential. There is an inherent desire for order and routine, sometimes excessive. Overdrawing on your reserves can have serious consequences.

Massage: Treat yourself to a massage or bodywork session as frequently as you can. Your tendency to muscular tension will be eased and soothed.

Hypnosis: This is a good way to get past constant mental chatter and activity, and fear and

SUPPORTIVE EXERCISES

You usually find goal-oriented exercise, such as weight training and competitive activities enjoyable, but you should guard against exercise becoming compulsive. There is also a need, however, to let go into more creative modes, so dance is an excellent form of exercise for you. Middle Eastern or Arabic dance styles, such as *Raqs Sharqi*, and Gabrielle Roth's "Five Elements" dance cycle are ideal.

apprehension. It bypasses the rational mind and helps achieve deep levels of relaxation.

BENEFICIAL HERBS

Tension-relievers: Especially good are wild oat, skullcap, and vervain. Lime blossom, cramp bark, and black cohosh relieve muscular tension. Also, see suggestions for the high resistance type.

Digestive-supporting: Bitter tonics (this is usually for a mixed or hematogenic color type) support your digestion and ensure you get a maximum uptake of nutrients.

Adaptogenics: Siberian ginseng, wild oat, and schisandra improve stamina and tone the adrenals.

THE GLANDULAR-EMOTIONAL IRIS

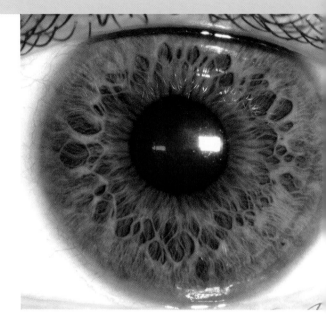

The glands central to this iris type are the endocrine organs, whose function is to regulate metabolic activity through the release of hormones.

Another term describing these people is polyglandular and this indicates that if one gland is functioning abnormally, others also may be affected. The glandular system works as a unit; the pituitary or master gland, in the brain, directs the rest elsewhere in the body. Many hormonal activities are triggered by signals from the pituitary.

Often called the "flower" or "daisy" type, the glandular-emotional iris structure is identified by the presence of lacunae (holes in the surface texture) in a ring around the collarette. It appears in all color types but in the hematogenic iris, the holes tend to be smaller.

The area immediately outside the collarette is known as the humoral zone, and refers to deep body fluids—blood, and lymph, or as the hormonal zone. Interrupted iris texture in this area suggests a potential for a disruption of hormone function.

CHARACTERISTIC TENDENCIES

These people are capable of tremendous energetic output, but require frequent periods of recuperation. After a day of unusual exertion, they will usually want to rest. They have a strong emotional side and wear their hearts on their sleeves. They can flow effortlessly between a wide range of emotional responses, but mood swings can be a problem. Open spaces in the iris also denote receptivity, and these people resonate readily with others, are great listeners, and are very creative.

Physiologically, these people may suffer from hormonal complaints The erratic functioning of the pituitary, thyroid, and adrenal glands and the pancreas, can portend problems with energy management. People of this type may be more vulnerable to menopausal difficulties, underactive thyroid, adrenal exhaustion, and type II diabetes, the latter being especially common in people of the mixed and hematogenic iris types.

A tendency early in life to hypoglycemia can warn of a later potential for diabetes if it is not addressed; an overactive thyroid can become underactive later; a tendency to hyperactivity of the adrenals may become chronic fatigue. Thus, unmanaged activity early in life can lead to exhaustion later. Work is needed to restore balance and moderation and this will prolong the life of the organs concerned.

Digestion is crucial in maintaining good operation of the hormonal glands, and taking bitter tonics to stimulate digestion will help achieve this.

Living with a Glandular-Emotional Constitution

Knowing what to eat, how to exercise, and what other lifestyle changes should be followed will help you to deal with your challenges, particularly regarding hormonal regulation.

DIETARY NEEDS

Food-combining: Refrain particularly from eating protein and carbohydrate together. This prevents overtaxing the pancreas. See also page 123.

Eat little and frequently: Small meals, eaten often, can help sustain energy. Choose fruit, dried fruit, nuts, oatcakes, rice cakes, hummus, and nut spreads.

THINGS TO AVOID

Sugars: Reduce consumption of refined and simple sugars like candies, chocolate, and cakes. These give energy, but it dissipates quickly.

A HEALTHY LIFESTYLE

Frequent breaks and rest: Variable iris texture implies changeable energy patterns. You need frequent breaks at work and plenty of rest. Avoid burning the candle at both ends, especially as you get older. Late nights must be balanced with wholesome food, exercise, and sleep.

BENEFICIAL HERBS

Improve erratic energy levels with herbal remedies. See pages 116–17 for instructions on preparing herbal teas and drinks.

Digestion-supporting: Bitter tonics, including gentian, the wormwood family, citrus peel, and Swedish bitters, stimulate digestion and absorption.

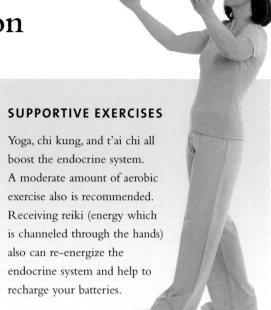

SUPPORTIVE EXERCISES

Yoga, chi kung, and t'ai chi all boost the endocrine system. A moderate amount of aerobic exercise also is recommended. Receiving reiki (energy which is channeled through the hands) also can re-energize the endocrine system and help to recharge your batteries.

Endocrine-supporting: For the pituitary gland, use dong quai, chaste tree berry, mugwort, ginkgo, and St John's Wort. For an underactive thyroid, take kelp, nettle, damiana, and oatseed. For an overactive thyroid, use bugle weed, valerian, skullcap, and oatseed. For the pancreas, take bitters, dandelion, burdock, fenugreek, garlic, and juniper berry. For the adrenals, use panax ginseng, Siberian ginseng, astragalus, oatseed, burdock, licorice, and borage. For male hormones, take ginseng, damiana, withania, oatseed, and sarsaparilla. For female hormones, use dong quai, chaste tree berry, cramp bark, partridge berry, black cohosh, ginger, and castor oil (on the skin).

THE GASTRIC IRIS

The gastric disposition is very similar to the glandular-emotional, of which it may be considered a subtype. The difference is that the lacunae in the gastric iris are inside the collarette, not just outside it. The effect is to expand the collarette toward the edge of the iris so that the space inside it is as great as, if not greater than, the portion of the iris outside it. Typically there also will be many smaller crypts inside the lacunae, especially at the collarette. The overall effect is much looser texture and darker shading inside the collarette than outside it.

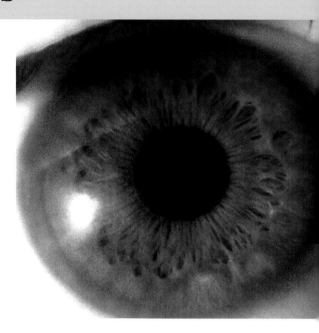

CHARACTERISTIC TENDENCIES

The emphasis for people of this type is on the gastrointestinal tract, and these people have a predisposition toward disturbances such as indigestion and acid stomach, bloating after eating, constipation, diverticulitis (inflammation of the lining of the gut), colitis, *dysbiosis*, and *candidosis* (disruption of natural gut bacteria and consequent overgrowth of the Candida albicans organism).

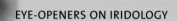

EYE-OPENERS ON IRIDOLOGY

CONSTIPATION People of this type can suffer from constipation and will benefit from herbal purgatives. Senna, cascara, dandelion, dock, and some varieties of aloe contain anthraquinones. Anthraquinones irritate and thus stimulate the smooth muscles of the bowel, causing an increase in peristalsis (the natural movement which pushes fecal matter).

Parasites are a common problem, and may be acquired easily, especially if gut health is not well maintained. The gastric type has a greater need to pay attention to the gut to avoid such problems.

In some schools this type is referred to as the "abdominal reservoir," implying that much is held in the stomach and intestines. This may be literal, as in constipation, but it also may be figurative, as in hanging on to emotions and awareness. Constipation often is associated with a tendency to hang on to the past. On the positive side, this pattern implies greater awareness of the emotional self and relying on "gut instincts."

Gastric people need to take care of their gastrointestinal tracts, and to be wary of becoming habituated to problems, for example, constipation. The chronic retention of toxic waste material in the gut can be the forerunner of many degenerative diseases, including colo-rectal cancer. Many of the suggestions given for the glandular iris type can be applied to the gastric disposition.

Living with a Gastric Constitution

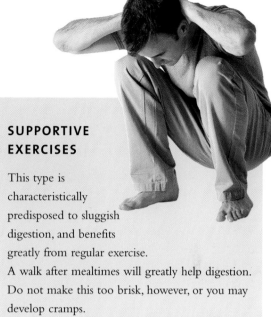

Eating the right foods and making other lifestyle changes will help you deal effectively with your challenges, particularly regarding digestion.

DIETARY NEEDS

Fiber: Eat plenty of whole grains, wholemeal bread, dried peas and beans, fruit, and vegetables.

Fruit: Eat plenty of fruit, both fresh and dried, but seek advice on dried fruit if you suspect you have a candida overgrowth. Prunes, figs, and prune juice are good remedies for constipation.

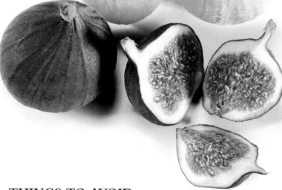

THINGS TO AVOID

Sugar and refined carbohydrates and fat: These provide only "empty" calories and are not supportive to the digestive system.

BENEFICIAL HERBS

Soothing: Slippery elm, marshmallow, licorice, linseed, and psyllium husks act as gentle laxatives, but also soothe and rebuild the gastrointestinal tract. These are taken as powders, using one heaped teaspoon mixed with a mug of water or juice, drunk once or twice a day. Other purgatives beneficial for this type are senna and cascara, which are taken as capsules or tinctures.

SUPPORTIVE EXERCISES

This type is characteristically predisposed to sluggish digestion, and benefits greatly from regular exercise. A walk after mealtimes will greatly help digestion. Do not make this too brisk, however, or you may develop cramps.

My favorite exercise for this type is the squat, which works on energetic principles, and may be considered a form of yoga.

To perform the squat, stand with your feet hip-width apart. You may need to hold onto the back of a chair as you gently lower yourself, bending your knees and keeping your feet flat on the ground. Try bouncing a little to ease yourself down, but do not rise onto the balls of your feet. If you can, go all the way down, flop forward over your knees, clasp your hands at the back of your neck, and gently pull your head down. Breathe deeply into the abdomen—this will stretch you even further. Bounce a little again, easing into the posture, and relaxing on the outbreath. Maintain the posture for two to five minutes. Rise slowly and arch your back a little to stretch out in the opposite direction. By compressing, and then stretching out the abdomen, you stimulate the internal organs in a gentle fashion.

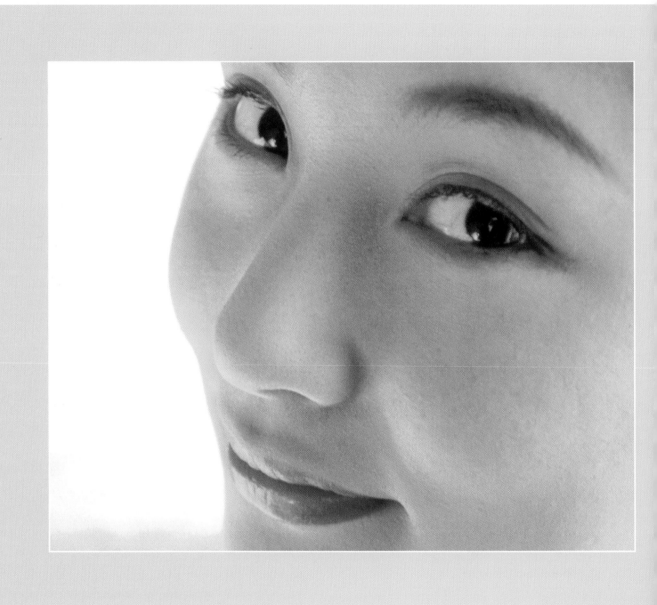

5

THE IRIS & ITS SIGNS

The true individuality of the iris is discovered in the deviations of structure and color that make up the unique iris pattern. This chapter explores those markings and what they might mean. You shouldn't rigidly interpret these signs as indications of disease. Signs in the iris are generally to be considered as genetically inherited markers for certain tendencies or predispositions. There may be up to 200 different signs in an iris, and we will explore ways of deciding how to determine if a sign is important or not. Not all signs are necessarily anchored to their topographical positions on the iris chart.

There are two types of signs: Topostabile signs are significant according to their position on the chart; topolabile signs are significant for their general appearance, and can occur anywhere on the chart. Structural signs are generally topostabile, showing a tendency within the field in which they are seen. Variations in the placement of the iris fibers are their defining characteristics.

Lacuna Types

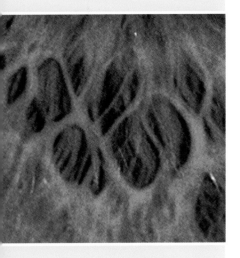

There are several types of lacuna (of which we will look at four), and they indicate areas where there is a need to restore and stimulate, improve blood flow, enhance lymphatic drainage, and boost the flow of energy.

CLOSED LACUNA

Completely encircled with a fibrous border so that it looks like a hole in the texture, a closed lacuna (see left) is regarded as a sign that one of your ancestors had a problem with the organ in that sector of the iris. A common example is a closed lacuna in the heart zone, which may show that an ancestor had heart disease or a heart attack. This does not mean you will have a heart attack, but you should be aware of the inherent weakness in the organ and avoid behavior that could exacerbate it.

OPEN LACUNA

A hole in the texture that does not have a complete border and that has a section on the same level as the surrounding iris tissue is an open lacuna. While it indicates a potentially more serious situation—it points to a condition that may not yet have occurred or that is in process—you can have more influence over its development. For example, if you have a recurrent chest complaint, you may have an open lacuna in your lung zone. The sign depicts a condition that needs to be healed. If you choose foods that strengthen the lungs and the immune system, such as garlic, onion, berries (for vitamin C and antioxidants), echinacea, wild cherry bark, elecampane, marshmallow, and licorice, you will improve your organs' defenses and possibly avoid passing on problems to the next generation. Using antibiotics to suppress a condition may store up trouble for later.

Another important aspect of both open and closed lacunae is the depth of the hole. The iris is composed of about four layers of fibers. Some holes only affect the surface layer, with plenty of fibers visible within them, while others penetrate to the deepest level, appearing darker or black.

Lacunae may assume a variety of different shapes, and there are slightly different interpretations for each variation. However, the principles listed above give a good general understanding of how to interpret them.

CRYPTS

A common example of a lacuna that penetrates to the deepest level of the iris is a crypt, which is small and diamond-shaped. Crypts are often found

SUGGESTED REMEDIES

 THERAPIES Hydrotherapy, castor oil packs

 DIET Foods to strengthen the lungs and the immune system: garlic, onion, berries (for vitamin C and antioxidants)

 HERBS Echinacea, elecampane, wild cherry bark, marshmallow, licorice

 EMOTIONS Vulnerability, changeability, or confusion; capitulation to the demands of others; self pity; lack of defenses or boundaries; inability to say "no"

around the intestinal zone, and are signs of the potential for degenerative conditions within the intestines, often involving parasite activity.

A smaller version of the crypt is the "defect of substance" marking. This is regarded as a sign for chronic degenerative conditions. These markings are small, black, pinprick holes that puncture to the deepest level. The smaller the hole, the more serious its significance may be.

Crypts and defect markings may frequently be spotted inside larger lacunae. An example of this is the honeycomb lacuna, where a bordered lesion contains a network of smaller holes. These are often seen in the digestive zone and are considered signs of parasitic infestation.

RAREFACTION

These are variations in fiber density. The fiber structure is looser, there may not be a specific fibrous boundary to the area, and the color appears darker. Less density and darker shading imply reduced resistance and lowered vitality. Rarefactions indicate organs in which problems may arise as a result of lowered immunity and insufficient self-cleansing.

LEARNING FROM LACUNAE

On the one hand, lacunae present opportunities for healing and for dispersing accumulated stress. They also point to receptivity, emotional honesty, creativity, and acceptance. On the other hand, they are warning signs, indicating reduced connective tissue strength leading to poor nourishment, drainage, immunity, and lowered local vitality and resistance; toxicity; parasite infestation; inherent organ weakness; ancestral disease patterns; insufficiency; and retention and accumulation, leading to cysts and tumors. They also can indicate vulnerability, emotional confusion, a tendency to capitulate to others, and self pity.

Try to assess whether a lacuna is open or closed and its depth. These structural signs will not change during your life. They may occasionally look different due to fluctuations in pupil size, but they remain the same size, depth, and in the same positions as when they crystallized in your eyes soon after you were born.

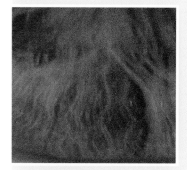

Open lacuna

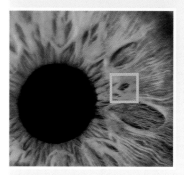

Crypt

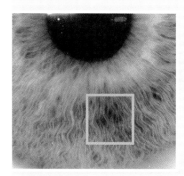

Rarefaction

Collarette Signs

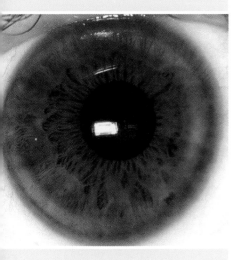

An important diagnostic tool, the collarette will tell you about your digestive tract and autonomic nervous system. A roughly circular structure around your pupil, about a third of the way out toward the edge of the iris, deviations in the collarette can have implications for the organs in the zone immediately adjacent.

Collarette signs have a variety of appearances. Below I discuss generally how to interpret and treat them. Bear in mind that the collarette is the reflex site for the autonomic nervous system, so consider the influence of the nervous system in any condition arising.

PROMINENT, WHITE, AND HYPERACTIVE
Irritable bowel syndrome and other stress-related disease may be apparent. Treatment isn't possible without addressing the causative factors, which could be nervous tension; reduced digestive efficiency due to weakening of the liver, gallbladder, and pancreas; and disturbed gastrointestinal immunity. Use herbs such as valerian, vervain, and skullcap to relax and soothe; deep breathing and yoga, such as the shoulderstand; and meditation, relaxation techniques, and visualizations.

THIN OR INVISIBLE
You need to stimulate digestion and the production of digestive enzymes to improve the absorption and distribution of nutrients, and guard against sluggishness. Use bitters, spices, and pungent foods such as garlic, ginger, and cayenne in your food.

EXPANDED
If there is a loose texture in the pupillary zone, there may be a tendency to atonal constipation: sluggish bowels due to lack of tone in the peristaltic muscles. Any protuberances or deep lacunae in the collarette warn of potential diverticular pockets or diverticulosis, in which fecal matter and parasitic infestation may be retained. Bowel cleanses should be used.

CONTRACTED
Constipation will be spasmodic. The need here is to release and relax. Use tinctures or teas containing wild yam and black cohosh, and gentle laxatives such as linseed, psyllium, and slippery elm taken as powders mixed with water or juice.

SUGGESTED REMEDIES

THERAPIES
White collarette deep breathing, yoga, meditation, relaxation techniques, visualization
Expanded collarette intensive bowel cleansing routines

DIET **Thin collarette** garlic, ginger, cayenne

HERBS **White collarette** valerian, vervain, skullcap
Thin collarette bitters, chilli, coriander, cumin, cardamom
Contracted collarette wild yam, black cohosh, linseed, psyllium, slippery elm

Fiber Types

Certain types suggest trauma and inflammation and symptoms may appear either physically or psychologically.

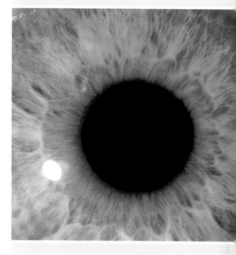

IRRITATION FIBER

A prominent, bright, or white fiber running from the collarette to the iris edge, it signifies irritation and reactivity in the organ represented in that portion of the iris (refer to the chart, pages 76–77). If it appears in the left eye at 15 minutes or the right at 45 minutes, it reveals a potential for stress-related heart disease. In a mixed iris an irritation fiber in the relevant location can show gallbladder problems.

TRANSVERSAL AND REFLEXIVE FIBERS

A transversal fiber runs across the grain of the iris, whereas a reflexive fiber starts off in the right direction but veers off. These are thought to indicate trauma or accidental damage. They also can indicate acute or chronic inflammation and potential tissue changes. Transversals may come in several patterns, including forked or "root-like" appearances, which are regarded as more serious. Look for the origin and destination of the transversal—these are the organs likely to be affected. An example of this is the so-called "spleen-heart" transversal, seen in the left iris, which is a sign for a possible risk of heart attack.

Check whether symptoms are physical or psychological and check the position of the fiber. A transversal in the liver field, for example, may mean suppression of anger, and you will need to address the emotional issues. Use treatments to decongest and cool the liver, such as bitter tonics and milk thistle tincture. Detoxification and enhancing immunity will better enable your body to rid itself of abnormal cells.

VASCULARIZATION

Each iris fiber is a microscopic vessel. Under stress, the vessel may engorge with blood and its outer sheath can split away, revealing a pink thread. These vascularizations heal with time, however, returning to a whitish appearance. Vascularization may be a sign of physical trauma affecting the organ indicated. A vascularized transversal may be a sign of a buried emotional trauma. Treatment takes a pacifying approach for trauma and inflammation, using the herbs listed (see right).

SUGGESTED REMEDIES

Transversal and reflexive fibers
THERAPIES Liver flush

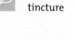

HERBS Bitter tonics, milk thistle tincture

EMOTIONS Work with suppressed anger or resentment

Vascularization
HERBS For trauma and healing wounds: St John's Wort, comfrey (external use only), marigold, arnica (external use only, except homeopathic pills), aloe vera
For soothing nerves: skullcap, vervain, passionflower

Furrow Types

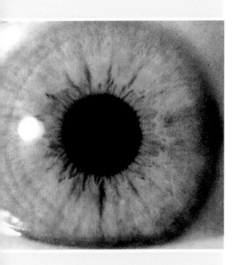

SUGGESTED REMEDIES

Contraction furrows

THERAPIES
Massage

EMOTIONS Nervous tension,
tendency to internalize stress,
a yearning for freedom, fear

Radial furrows

THERAPIES
Bowel cleansing program

Contraction and radial furrows (see left) are very common in the self-protective iris, where we see these signs in abundance.

CONTRACTION FURROWS

These look like ripples in the surface of the iris and can be partial or plentiful, extending around the iris disc in a concentric pattern. Sometimes also called "nerve rings," they are signs of nervous tension and a tendency to internalize stress. They also imply that you use nutritional energy up quickly, need to eat carefully and regularly, and not become exhausted.

Look for breaks in the rings: these are the points where stress may be causing problems. However, in a dense iris with few other structural signs, they may be the only opportunities for the release of stress, and are possibly similar in meaning to lacunae or rarefactions in a less dense iris.

Contraction furrows can imply a sense of being imprisoned in the body and can conceal a yearning for physical and emotional freedom, which is nonetheless frightening, as it involves the dissolution of one's defenses.

RADIAL FURROWS

Radial furrows come in two forms: major radials start at the pupil edge and cut through the collarette as it points toward the outer iris edge; minor radials start at the collarette. Major radials imply a weakening of the autonomic nerve system. Radials are both a sign of potential for toxic leakage from a congested bowel and a sign of nerve weakness, particularly affecting the gastrointestinal tract, but also the radial zone in which they appear (consult the iris chart, pages 76–77).

If constipated bowels are diagnosed, cleansing and regenerating them may show up in the radials "emptying" themselves of toxic material, becoming clearer and lighter. If nerve weakness is thought to be the problem, you need to support, tone, and nourish the nerves (see the self-protective type, pages 46–47).

Treatment for contraction and radial furrows

Massage is highly effective for contraction furrows. As these furrows also suggest increased utilization of nutrients, checking for and treating digestive weaknesses is important. For radial furrows, see the self-protective type, pages 46–47 for further information. If furrows have a congested appearance (look dark and full) consider a bowel cleansing program.

Pigment Signs

Pigment signs are regarded as the opposite to lacunae in terms of meaning. Whereas lacunae signify insufficiency, pigment signifies excess, concentration, and crystallization.

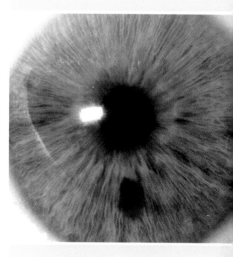

LEARNING FROM YOUR PIGMENTATION

Pigmentation of the whole iris determines constitutional type but spots or flecks of pigment or sections of different color also can occur in the iris. Pigment signs are usually deposits in the anterior border layer, a transparent film that covers the iris. Pigments indicate an accumulation of potentially toxic pollutants or metabolic wastes; a sluggishness or blockage of energy in affected organs or systems; a tendency to excess and crystallization, such as gallstones or kidney stones; tissue changes (shown by darker colors); a reduced flow of digestive enzymes; and protection of organs from excess stimulation by heat or light.

Pigments indicate resistance, self-protection, repression of emotions, obsessive thoughts and fears, an analytical or intellectual nature, secrecy, passion, aggression, insight, organizational abilities, and a visual nature.

Treatment for pigment signs

Use treatments that disperse accumulations and remove blockages, such as deep-tissue detoxification and therapies that move energy—polarity therapy, shiatsu, or acupuncture. Treatments that break up deposits, such as packs and poultices (see pages 108–9), can be applied to sites of cysts, polyps, tumors, calcification, pain, stiffness, and inflammation.

CLASSIFYING PIGMENTS

Each color has affinities with certain organs or systems (see chart overleaf). Pigment spots are usually interpreted according to color and appearance, showing which organ may be affected, and are topolabile (can occur anywhere on the iris chart); however, it may be important to note their position on the chart. Other pigment signs are the central and sectoral heterochromia. A central heterochromia is a different color in the middle and a sectoral heterochromia is a section of a different color. These appearances are topostabile—they affect the organs in that iris sector. For example, a central heterochromia highlights the digestive tract.

SUGGESTED REMEDIES

THERAPIES Deep-tissue detoxification, polarity therapy, shiatsu, acupuncture, castor oil packs

EMOTIONS Work on freeing your mind from unproductive thought patterns

PIGMENT DIFFERENTIATION CHART

Color	Organ	Description and interpretation
Straw yellow	Kidneys	Usually found as diffuse pigment around the collarette and humoral zone, and in flocculations and plaques throughout the ciliary zone. Can indicate bowel toxicity due to poor breakdown of animal proteins, and resultant stress on kidneys. Amplifies hyperacidic type.
Bright yellow Yellow ocher	Liver/Gallbladder	Found as isolated spots or patches inside and outside the collarette, and as central heterochromia and in plaques and flocculations. The more concentrated the color, the more the diathesis moves toward the gallbladder. Liver congestion and sluggishness (topolabile), intolerance to rich, fatty foods (dairy), difficulty with fat metabolism, and biliary dysfunction.
Orange Red orange	Pancreas	Found as spots and patches throughout the iris and as central heterochromia. Sometimes have a grainy or patchy appearance. Topolablile signs for pancreatic dysfunction, both endocrine (hypoglycemia, diabetes), and exocrine (provision of digestive enzymes). Care needed with proteins and carbohydrates, food combining recommended, and avoidance of refined sugars.
Bright red	Stomach	Patches and spots usually found within the stomach zone, often very small. Disturbances of stomach enzymes and secretions. Possibility of ulceration or malignancy.
Red brown Brown Dark brown	Liver/Colon	Patches, spots, central heterochromia, sectoral heterochromia. Also red-brown "snuff" pigments (ferrous chromatosis) in humoral zone. Disturbances of liver function, constipation, autointoxication. Very dark brown/black pigment depicts immune compromise and chronic lymphatic congestion.

CHANGING COLORS

Pigment signs are often influenced by your state of health. If your eyes appear greener when you are unwell, you may have an increase of yellow or brown pigment, implying problems with the liver or bowel. These may appear to clear up once you return to normal health. However, pigments are largely genetically determined and therefore not so subject to change as many would like to think. Significant change is usually only possible with long-term, intensive healing work.

Psychologically, pigment shows considerable mental activity and analysis. The darker the pigment, the greater the tendency to brooding and obsessiveness. Those with a scattering of dark brown or black spots (called tar pigments) frequently need help escaping from their thoughts. This tendency may be a cause of serious disturbance or suppression, particularly of immunity. However, when these people are in balance they are great intellectuals, scientists, and analysts.

Lymphatic Rosary

This is a ring of distinct white spots, sometimes in couplets, around the outer edge of the iris. It may be complete or partial.

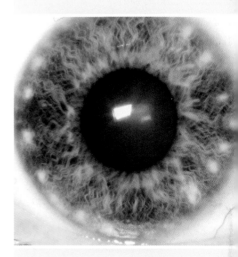

In its complete form the lymphatic rosary is referred to as the hydrogenoid or exudative diathesis. This is a subtype of the blue-eyed constitution. However, these spots also may be seen in brown eyes, where they are pigmented. In the complete form, the spots are bright white or cream-colored. The whiteness signifies hyper-reactivity and an over-enthusiastic immune system. Indeed, allergy may be defined as an over-active immune system, which mounts defensive reactions against ordinary, usually harmless, substances. Behind this reactivity there will often be an overloading of the tissues, specifically connective tissue and lymphatic tissue.

A lymphatic rosary indicates the possibility of congestion and overloading of the lymphatic channels, the body's internal drainage system, and of the mucous membranes. This sign may show a predisposition to conditions affecting the upper respiratory tract, including allergic conditions such as hay fever or rhinitis; phlegm and post-nasal drip; tonsillitis; and swollen glands around the neck, throat, armpits, and groin.

A person with a complete ring may tend toward the psychological traits of perfectionism, a dislike of conflict, and a strong desire to control his or her environment. When healthy, this person may be a creator of beautiful environments, a diplomat, or a peacemaker. He or she may like to clean and tidy, which can sometimes be obsessive. When sick or out of balance, this person may be controlling and "houseproud."

Treatment for the lymphatic rosary

Use the following herbs as tinctures or teas to stimulate lymphatic cleansing and to relieve the burden on mucous membranes: cleavers, mullein, nettle, yellow dock, elder, and echinacea. Herbs to soothe mucous membranes and reduce allergic reaction are plantain (ribwort), mullein, marshmallow, and licorice. Advanced lymphatic cleansers are poke root, lobelia, and chaparral tinctures. The latter are not advised without professional support. It is necessary to use more gentle cleansers as a preparation before taking these herbs, to avoid possible side effects. Exercise and deep breathing keep lymph moving.

SUGGESTED REMEDIES

 HERBS Stimulate lymph: cleavers, mullein, nettle, yellow dock, elder, echinacea. Soothe mucous membranes and reduce allergic reaction: plantain (ribwort), mullein, marshmallow, licorice

 EMOTIONS Work on self-acceptance and acceptance of others, try not to over-control

Clouds, Wisps, and Plaques

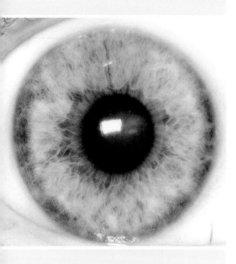

Cloudiness over the iris indicates an accumulation of metabolic acidic wastes that your body is unable to discharge.

This shows a predisposition to gout and arthritis, which are brought about by the irritation of connective tissue by retained acidic residues. Such acid wastes also can become irritating to the heart and may portend circulatory disturbances. Your kidneys may be at risk, as they are responsible for discharging these waste substances. Your liver, too, has a role in metabolizing uric acid, and should be investigated.

Sometimes the clouds may bear some pigment. A wash of straw yellow is common, giving the eyes a greenish appearance. In this case, the kidneys may be under stress, particularly from incompletely digested protein residues entering the blood from a congested colon. As well as supporting the kidneys, the bowels should be cleansed.

Your skin, which discharges uric acid through perspiration, may need attention. People who have clouds, wisps, and plaques in their irides hold a lot in, both physiologically and emotionally, and sometimes feel like they can't take on anything else. They need to work on letting things go emotionally. They can be resistant to therapy, since they feel that taking this on is burdensome. The presence of a scurf rim amplifies the tendencies of this hyperacidic type, and increases the tendency to hold things in.

Treatment for clouds, wisps, and plaques

Drink plenty of water to flush out and buffer the acids. Adopt an alkaline diet, with low or no salt (excess salt will result in the body retaining water to buffer the sodium). Avoid red meat, pork, and pig products (all high in uric acid), excessive alcohol, coffee, and some grain foods, especially wheat. Eat plenty of fresh fruits and vegetables and drink fresh juices. A rough guide for an alkaline diet is 60 percent fresh fruits and vegetables and 40 percent split between proteins, carbohydrates, and fats. In the summer the proportions can be changed to 80/20.

To remove uric acid, alkalize the blood, and improve kidney function, include the following herbs: celery seed, wild carrot, nettle, parsley piert, bearberry, buchu, dandelion, and corn silk. Add marshmallow root or leaf to reduce irritation to mucous membranes. Horsetail strengthens the bladder. All of these herbs can be taken as teas or tinctures.

SUGGESTED REMEDIES

 DIET Lots of water; alkaline diet; low or no salt; eat plenty of fresh fruits and vegetables and juices. Avoid red meat, pork, bacon and ham; alcohol and coffee, and grain foods, especially wheat

 HERBS Celery seed, wild carrot, nettle, parsley piert, bearberry, buchu, dandelion, corn silk, marshmallow root or leaf, horsetail

 EMOTIONS Try to let difficult feelings go

The Scurf Rim

A dark band at the outer edge of the iris, this often can be seen clearly in pale blue eyes without the aid of a magnifier. It is very common to the hyperacidic type and also to the rheumatic type (see pages 24–25 on the Blue Iris).

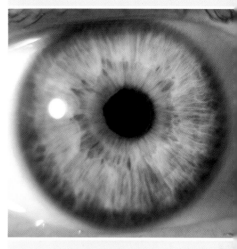

This sign indicates that the skin is under-active, is not discharging well, and may become overloaded and congested. This may manifest in the form of an outbreak—eczema, psoriasis, acne, or sensitivity, itchiness, and dryness.

The outer zone of the iris is the zone of elimination: darkness or rarefaction (see the earlier section on structural signs) in this zone depict poor elimination, which results in a buildup and overloading of toxins, and must be tackled by a suitable therapeutic program. Stimulating the skin also will relieve pressure on the kidneys, which may be struggling to cope with excessive elimination. Psychologically, there is a tendency to hold in emotions, especially irritation and anger, suppression of which may be a direct cause of skin outbreaks, and should form part of the treatment.

The skin is our physical interface with the environment, and skin eruptions tend to imply some suppression of feelings concerning our interactions with the world and others. We may not express this verbally or behaviorally, but our system may express it in an outbreak of some kind, possibly on our skin. Examine feelings of anger or resentment and try to come to terms with them. Work on feeling safe. Skin problems also can imply a lack of trust of others and an inability to express negative feelings.

SUGGESTED REMEDIES

 THERAPIES Dry skin brushing, hydrotherapy

 HERBS Mountain grape root, burdock, elderflower, peppermint, spearmint, yarrow, ginger

 EMOTIONS Work on self-expression and feeling safe

Treatment for the scurf rim

Use dry skin brushing or other forms of exfoliation. Also, hydrotherapy—the use of hot and cold water—stimulates the skin, as do saunas, steam baths, and Turkish baths. Don't forget to use the cold plunge. If you have circulatory problems, ask a health professional what course of action would be appropriate.

Mountain grape root and burdock are both blood cleansing herbs that work on the liver and kidneys and have a special affinity with the skin. Elderflower, peppermint or spearmint, and yarrow and ginger are good to promote perspiration. These herbs are best taken as teas.

The Cholesterol Ring

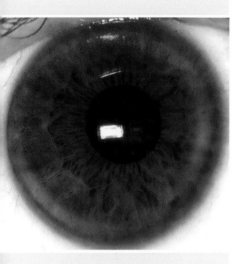

This is also called the lipemic ring (referring to blood fats), the sodium ring (referring to blood composition), or the arcus senilis ("the arc of old age").

This is a medically recognized sign that appears in the cornea, not the iris, although it obscures the outer ring of the iris. It is a sign of the tendency to develop high blood fats.

This ring consists of an opaque white circle around the outer zone of the iris. It builds up in the eye slowly over time, generally beginning as a partial ring or arc, and gradually expanding to complete the ring. Although it is a medically recognized sign for the presence of high blood fats (including cholesterol), many doctors also consider that it is a natural sign of old age. When it appears in the upper segment of the iris, it portends possible memory problems, or at the most extreme, a stroke or senile dementia. It also indicates insufficient nourishment and oxygenation of the cerebral circulation, leading to poor function of the brain. In its complete ring-form it also warns of possible coronary arterial blockage, leading to heart failure.

It is much more common in people with pure dark brown irides (hematogenic) than the other two constitutional types; however, it can occur in all types. Because it is not a sign seen from birth, it is assumed to be evidence of an acquired condition. However, it is also considered to portray a genetic predisposition to difficulty with regulating blood fats. It can begin to appear as early as the mid-twenties, but more usually is first seen as a faint, translucent hazy ring between the ages of 40 and 50, and if nothing is done to reverse it, it continues to develop.

An early symptom associated with the sign is cold extremities, particularly the feet, and this more specifically if the arc is in the lower portion of the iris. It is a matter of fat-laden blood being too thick to penetrate the narrow peripheral vessels.

Cholesterol levels

People with this sign are advised to check their cholesterol levels regularly and change their diets. This is a precautionary measure: blood fats may prove to be within normal limits, but this sign can appear in advance of the clinical problem being obvious.

This sign can indicate both athero- and arteriosclerosis. The former is the deposition of fats onto the arterial walls, and the consequent narrowing

SUGGESTED REMEDIES

 DIET Low-fat, low-salt; naturopathic liver flush

 HERBS Garlic, artichoke leaf, motherwort, hawthorn, cayenne, ginger, ginkgo, red clover

 EMOTIONS Do not be dogmatic or over-identified with your opinions, cultivate flexibility of mind

of the vessels. The latter is hardening of the arteries, due to deposition of calcium and sodium—hence the term "sodium ring." This sign also may be acquired through excessive salt consumption, and shows how excess sodium, cholesterol, and calcium contribute to the hardening of the tissues in which they settle.

People with this sign may appear quite stubborn, resist change, and be set in their ways. However, they also may be described as idealistic and determined, and see their resistance as a reluctance to have their ideals and beliefs challenged or diluted in any way. They make good campaigners for any cause. Regarding emotions, they need to guard against a tendency to be dogmatic or over-identified with their own opinions.

Treatment for the cholesterol ring

A low-fat, low-salt diet must be followed. Frequent efforts should be made to care for and maintain the liver—the naturopathic liver flush (see page 115) is very effective.

Garlic, artichoke leaf, and motherwort help to lower cholesterol; hawthorn strengthens circulatory vessels and protects the heart; cayenne and ginger stimulate circulation; and ginkgo and red clover thin the blood. These herbs should be taken as teas or tinctures, except garlic, which should be eaten whole and raw as a food.

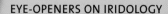

EYE-OPENERS ON IRIDOLOGY

CHOLESTEROL RING This does not necessarily mean that you have a high-fat diet. One man I saw with this sign had been a vegan for 13 years. His cholesterol level was found to be more than 9 (normal is below 5). He was under enormous stress, which can alter the balance of HDL and LDL (good and bad) cholesterol. Also, there is an element of inheritance with this sign. Treatment needs to work on the liver to reverse and balance this condition, as it is chiefly the liver that metabolizes fats. Lifestyle and psychological issues—especially stress—also need to be addressed.

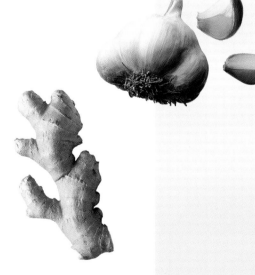

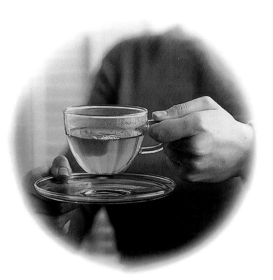

The Dyscratic Overlay

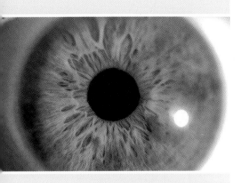

Dyscrasia is a medical term meaning disturbance through toxic overloading of the blood, lymph, and connective tissue.

The dyscratic overlay is a buildup of pigments of different colors and is considered to be an acquired condition, accumulating as life progresses, and receding to some extent when appropriate measures are taken.

Why do some people acquire dyscrasia and not others? It seems that there is a genetic element. People with this tendency may be at increased risk of liver, gallbladder, and pancreatic disease (including diabetes); inflammatory joint and connective tissue diseases (rheumatism and arthritis); bowel disorders; and, if conditions persist, malignancies.

Dyscrasia often goes along with hyperacidic cloudiness—the clouds may bear the pigmentation. People with this pattern may feel burdened and have persistent negative thought patterns. Work on discarding negativity.

Treatment for the dyscratic overlay
Undertake frequent cleansing and detoxifying periods—maybe three or four times a year—to maintain good tissue cleanliness, taking in the bowels, kidneys, liver, and lymphatics. A raw food diet or juice fasts should be the basis of this practice for five to seven days. Intoxicating influences should be strictly avoided.

SUGGESTED REMEDIES

 THERAPIES Liver flush, kidney flush

 DIET Raw foods, juices, avoid simple sugars, saturated fats

 EMOTIONS Let go of negative thought habits

The Anemia Ring

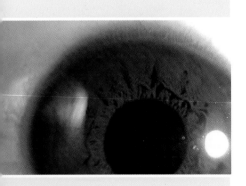

This appears as a fuzzy edge to the iris in the upper and/or lower sectors. It is caused by the sclera, or white of the eye, invading the iris, thus blurring the edge.

This ring indicates a tendency to cold extremities—failure of the blood to oxygenate or nourish the peripheral tissues. In the cerebral region, this leads to problems with memory and mental function, similar to those described for the cholesterol ring. When in an advanced state, it can signify a more general anemic condition.

The Venous Ring

A blue ring around the outer edge of the iris shows sluggishness and congestion of the venous circulation, that is the vessels that carry blood back to the heart.

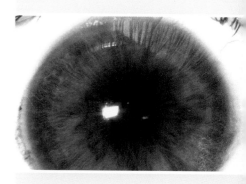

This results in poor elimination of carbon dioxide and acid wastes, as the venous blood has problems returning to the heart and lungs to discharge the wastes and become re-oxygenated. As a consequence, this leads to poor oxygenation of tissues in the anabolic part of the cycle.

This sign is seen most frequently in the hematogenic iris, where it amplifies constitutional concerns, but it is found in all iris types.

Treatment for the venous ring

The circulation needs to be stimulated and blood moved more efficiently. Inverted yoga postures and the use of slant-boards or equipment that enables you to reverse your normal gravitational direction are effective.

Garlic, ginger, and cayenne stimulate and cleanse the blood and circulation; red clover thins and cleanses the blood; hawthorn improves the elasticity of vessels; and horse chestnut is effective for varicose veins, including hemorrhoids, which often accompany this condition. These herbs should be taken as tinctures.

SUGGESTED REMEDIES

 HERBS Garlic, cayenne, ginger, red clover, hawthorn, horse chestnut

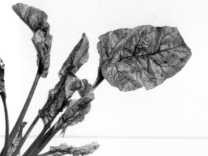

Treatment for the anemia ring

Eat foods that nourish the blood, such as dark green vegetables, beetroot and beetroot greens, and spinach; red fruits (high in antioxidants for blood cleansing); sprouted alfalfa seeds; and spirulina, chlorella, and other chlorophyll-rich foods (chlorophyll is chemically similar to hemoglobin).

Ginger, cayenne, and ginkgo improve blood flow to the extremities. Also, include herbs high in iron: devil's claw, yellow dock, raspberry leaf, and bilberry. These are taken as tinctures, although cayenne is used as a powder. Mix half a teaspoon with juice, or take two to three capsules daily.

SUGGESTED REMEDIES

 DIET Dark green vegetables, beetroot, red fruits, alfalfa, spirulina, chlorella

 HERBS Ginger, ginkgo, devil's claw, yellow dock, raspberry leaf, bilberry, cayenne powder

 EMOTIONS: Work on self-esteem and affirmation

Pupil Size & Shape

Sympathetic and parasympathetic nerve impulses control pupil size and shape deviations inform about the nervous system.

A permanently large pupil can indicate a person who has a tendency to adrenal hyperactivity, is always on the go, and who is quite sociable, but who finds it difficult to shut down. Extreme expansion of the pupils portends adrenal exhaustion and chronic fatigue. A permanently contracted pupil may indicate that a person is introverted, generally sluggish, has slow reactions, and lacks enthusiasm. When the sympathetic nervous system is weak, the parasympathetic is dominant, and vice versa. Treatment should work to moderate the dominant system and strengthen the weaker system.

Occasionally a person may have pupils of differing sizes (anisocoria). This can indicate a family history of syphilis, diphtheria, or meningitis, which may have compromised his or her nervous system and immune system.

Generally, deviations in any of the circular structures of the iris will reveal information about the nervous system (see page 85). The pupil may have areas of flatness around its circumference and the adjacent iris sector may show evidence of problems in the organ represented in that sector, so consult the iris chart (see pages 76–77) for more information. If a problem exists, consider the possibility that nerve supply may be involved, perhaps originating in a misalignment of the spine.

Spinal map

You can use the pupil margin as a map of the spine. Divide each pupil in half by drawing a line from top to bottom. Each half represents the spinal column, with the cervical spine at the top, the thoracic in the midsection, and the lumbar and sacral vertebrae in the lower segment, in each half. A spinal misalignment may be assumed from any section that is flattened (see above): simply estimate which area of the spine is involved. If the same flatness is in both pupils, the indication is reinforced.

PUPIL

RIGHT IRIS **LEFT IRIS**

KEY

Cervical spine (7 vertebrae)

Thoracic spine (12 vertebrae)

Lumbar spine (5 vertebrae)

Sacrum and coccyx

Psychological Interpretations

Indications in the iris also may be emotionally or psychologically significant, rather than physically or physiologically.

The following is a brief overview of psychological interpretations for different types of signs in the iris and the issues they highlight. However, there is not space in this book to explore this application of iridology in detail. If you would like to research these levels further, you should seek professional guidance and advice.

PSYCHOLOGICAL INTERPRETATIONS

Signs	Interpretation
Digestive signs (concentric zones 1 and 2)	Self-nourishment and the willingness (or not) to give and receive unconditional love; a yearning for a love that can never be satisfied due to a lack of belief that one deserves it or is capable of receiving it; eating disorders; an energetic connection to the earth.
Kidney and pelvic signs (bottom or ventral sector)	Self-determination and individuation; your creative potential; self-confidence; the role of fear in your upbringing, whether of punishment or of not being well-supported or appreciated; conditional love—striving to achieve in order to prove worthiness.
Liver, gallbladder, pancreas, and spleen signs (20 minutes and 40 minutes)	Anger, resentment, or frustration, and expressing these emotions; depression; capitulation to the demands of others (lacunae or rarefaction); boastful self-confidence that masks low self-esteem (pigment); perfectionism; assertiveness.
Lung signs (temporal sectors)	The ability (or not) to develop intimate relationships; an ability to share, expand toward others, and receive their expansion toward you; willingness to nourish yourself emotionally and physically (oxygen is a primary nutrient).
Heart and throat signs (nasal sectors, heart reflexes: left, 15 minutes and right, 45 minutes)	Honest expression; grief and yearning for union, both universal and human; isolation and separation; the ability or not to open up to life with joy and abandon.
Head area signs (top or frontal sector)	Depression, melancholy, moodiness (a lacuna at the pituitary/hypothalamus reflex can indicate Seasonal Affective Disorder (SAD) syndrome); preoccupation and obsession (pigments and radial furrows); spiritual dimension—a lacuna can signify spiritual opening or revelation, psychic abilities, or a strong religious or spiritual direction, often arrived at after emotional or psychological difficulty.

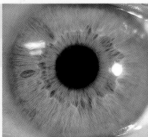

Stomach halo in the digestive zone

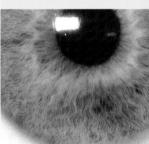

Rarefaction in the kidney zone

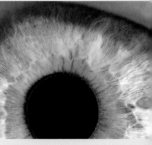

Crypt in the heart zone

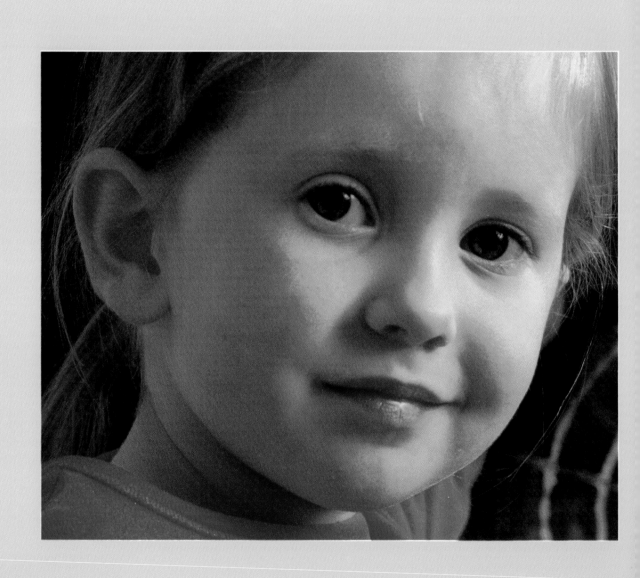

6

IRIS ZONES
& CHARTS

The iris chart breaks down the small disk of the iris into zones that give finely tuned information about the organs that fall within the zones. It is important to grasp the basic principles of iridology before you try and diagnose problems with individual organs or specific diseases. It is useful to have on hand a medical dictionary and a book on anatomy when studying the iris chart. When looking at your own eyes, you can observe the presence of signs and their positions and begin to ask yourself relevant questions. Wait until you have read chapter seven, however, before forming opinions about any problems you may have. Reading the chart is not the same as conducting a full assessment. Also, bear in mind that when you look at your eyes in a mirror, you are seeing a reverse image and need to calculate the correct positions.

CONCENTRIC ZONES OF THE IRIS

The concentric zones of the iris can tell us about our energy and health patterns.

The iris zones act as a flow chart, describing our tendencies in the absorption, digestion, distribution, and utilization of energy (food). It also reveals our ability to eliminate unused or toxic elements. The flow works from the center (pupil) outward.

Iris Zones

The rings of the iris are divided into four zones. The first one contains the stomach and intestinal rings; the second zone is the humoral; the third zone is utilization and the fourth zone is elimination.

PUPIL

Actually a gap or a lumen, you can think of the pupil as the unformed essence of a person. As we saw on page 68, a small pupil is a sign of withdrawal and secrecy, while a large pupil reflects an expansive, outward-going person. It is a matter of degree, and any extreme represents imbalance. A withdrawn person denies him- or herself contact with the world, and therefore misses out on the learning opportunities available through contact. An over-expansive type runs the risk of becoming exhausted, of not keeping enough in reserve.

PUPILLARY RUFF

This is also known as the inner pupil border (IPB), the neurasthenic ring, and the ring of absorption. It is the first point of contact of the pupil with

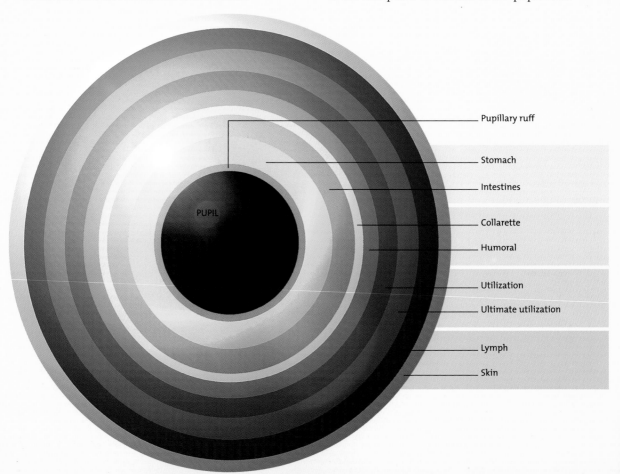

PUPIL

Pupillary ruff

Stomach

Intestines

Collarette

Humoral

Utilization

Ultimate utilization

Lymph

Skin

physical reality and describes how we react to and digest our experiences. This structure is minute, and you have to look hard to see it with a magnifier. It appears as an orange or red-brown ruff bordering the inner edge of the iris (see page 18 for a discussion of its anatomy).

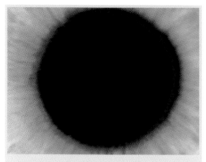

PUPILLARY RUFF This is a thin orange/red-brown ring around the inner edge of the iris.

• **A thick pupillary ruff** reflects a person who greets the challenges of life with enthusiasm, possibly even aggression, and who is outwardly focused in the physical world, but who may lack appreciation for the subtler, finer energies.

• **A thin pupillary ruff** indicates a person who shies away from life's challenges and may be quite timid. This person may find the harshness of the physical world overwhelming and can be hypersensitive.

It is normal for the pupillary ruff to be of varying thickness, usually split between thicker and thinner sections on a slightly diagonal, longitudinal axis. A specialist can read any variations in the sections and gain information about the central nervous system and how it is influenced by possible stresses on the spine. It should be possible to pinpoint the exact vertebrae involved, and make a diagnosis about the nerve supply to the organs indicated.

THE FOUR MAJOR ZONES OF THE IRIS
1st major zone: stomach and intestinal rings
This is also known as the pupillary or nutritive zone.

Stomach ring The next circular zone after the pupillary ruff, this

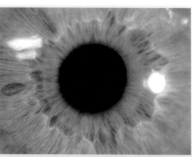

STOMACH HALO This appears as a regular whitish ring directly around the pupil.

can be seen as a regular, whitish halo just around the pupil. It generally reflects the position of the sphincter muscle, which lies beneath it in the iris body, and it can be seen clearly in some blue or pale mixed eyes.

The color of the stomach ring is important. Bright whiteness suggests over-reactivity; in this case, the tendency to produce too much hydrochloric acid and a disposition to gastric ulcers. It also may result in discomfort and reflux, especially if the valve at the top of the stomach, which prevents the contents of the stomach from re-entering the esophagus, is weak or has been weakened by a diet with too many carbohydrates and rich foods, and a tendency to over-eating. An incompetent valve is referred to as a hiatus hernia. The valve may be checked in the iris for signs of weakness (see the iris chart on pages 76–77).

A gray or muddy-looking stomach ring is an indication of a sluggish supply of digestive secretions from the stomach, and consequent failure to digest food properly. A normal stomach ring is not too dark, not too bright. Don't worry if you can't see yours. It is usually not visible in brown eyes and also is not visible in all blue eyes.

Intestinal ring This occurs immediately around the stomach ring. It is bordered on the other side by the collarette, which typically takes a varied course, and is rarely perfectly circular. The ins and outs of the collarette graphically describe the condition of the intestines. Areas of distension can indicate constipation, and an environment in which toxic and degenerative conditions are able to take hold. Conversely, where the collarette draws in, there can be strictures or spasmodic conditions affecting the intestines. The collarette also can be partially expanded, where it seems to invade the space of another organ. This can indicate consequences for that organ, which may be under pressure from a congested bowel. The intestinal ring also includes the sections of the small intestine. See page 78 for more information.

Humoral or assimilation zone

The zone of the deep body fluids, its position just outside the digestive reflexes gives it special significance for the way food is taken up and transported by the blood vessels surrounding the small intestine, and for the portal system—the blood flow into the liver and spleen, which is essential for processing nutriment. Another name for this zone is that of transportation and distribution. As we saw with the glandular-emotional iris (see pages 48–49), this region is also important for hormones, which also are transported by the blood.

There may be implications, too, for gastro-intestinal immunity. The mesenteric lymphatic vessels function here. There is a lot of lymph tissue around the gastrointestinal organs, because any area of the body open to outside influences must be defended against disease-causing organisms. The immune system regards anything entering the body as potentially harmful and monitors it all. Lymph tissue is present also in the mouth and throat (tonsils, adenoids), lungs (axillary nodes under the armpits), and groin (inguinal nodes).

Congestive appearances in the humoral zone may affect digestion and absorption, hormone function, and immunity.

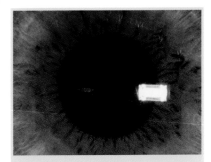

HUMORAL ZONE This is well-displayed in this mixed iris, in the band of orange-brown pigment flaring out from the collarette.

2nd major zone: utilization

This is composed of the zones of utilization and ultimate utilization.

Utilization zone: This zone concerns the body's use of nutriment. Here we find most of the major organs outside of the digestive tract, for example, the liver, kidneys, bladder, spleen, brain, and lungs. These are the organs that take up the energy from food and use it to keep us going. Having ingested, broken down, and distributed food, the body now puts it to work. Interruptions or congestive appearances in this field suggest a poor movement of nutritional energy throughout the system.

Ultimate utilization zone: This zone describes the musculo-skeletal system. The skeleton is also a store of minerals, especially calcium, for future use. Signs of weakness can indicate a tendency to mineral deficiency, possibly osteoporosis. White, inflammatory, or congestive signs may indicate arthritic or rheumatic disease.

3rd major zone: elimination

This consists of the lymph and skin zones. From it we can deduce how effectively the system discharges residues and metabolic waste products. A person whose zone is dark has difficulty in eliminating toxins and other residues, and his or her system retains this material unless efforts are made to overcome this tendency.

Lymph zone: This contains one of the major signs of the iris, the lymphatic rosary (see page 61).

Skin zone: While skin inflam-mation such as eczema has a stress component, it is also can be caused by a failure to eliminate. When the skin zone is dark we call it the scurf rim (see page 63).

THE IRIS REFLEX CHART

The concept that one part of the body contains clues about the rest of the system is not unique to iridology. Reflexology and Chinese face reading are two other well-known systems, both of which include a reflex pattern, in which the feet and the hands, or the face contain allotted points relating to all the other organs of the body. The first iris chart was produced by Ignatz von Peczely in the mid 19th century, and this forms the basis upon which most charts are drawn up. Von Peczely's chart has many of the organs in the same places that iridologists still recognize today.

Over the years, there have been many different versions of iris charts. Most of these agree on the basic positions, with differences mainly in the amount of detail shown.

The German iridologist and researcher, Joseph Angerer, produced one of the most detailed charts. His research led him to break down the iris into smaller reflex zones that give detailed information about the organs and their individual parts. However, without microscopy it can be difficult to differentiate the minutiae of such a chart, so most iridologists choose something a little less detailed. One of the most influential and well-known charts is Bernard Jensen's, and many modern charts have been developed from his.

The chart presented overleaf has been drawn up to reflect the major current trends in iris topography, while at the same time remaining simple and readable, not overcrowded, and yet with enough detail to enable quite a precise reading.

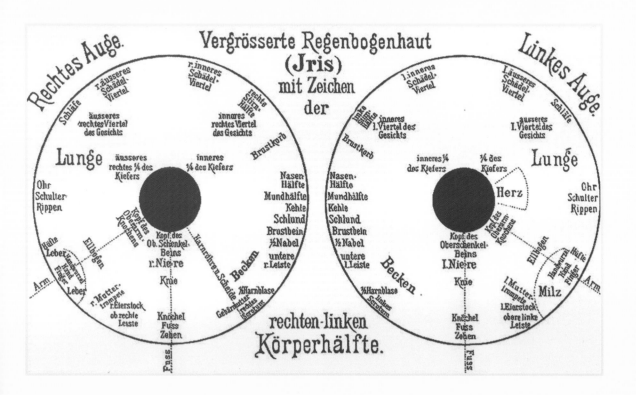

WORKING WITH THE CHART

HOW TO LOOK AT THE CHART

You can look at it from the front, as though you are facing the body. or from the top down, i.e., through the central lumen of the human body, as if you are traveling through the gastrointestinal tract. Taking the view from the front, you can see some basic correspondences: the brain is at the top, the lungs on each side, the liver mainly on the right, the spleen on the left, and the heart mainly on the left, but with a reflex site on the right, too. Some of these observations reflect the embryological development of the body.

When looking at the chart, remember it is as if you are looking at an individual, so the left eye will be to your right. The convention is to use positions of the clock to locate the organs, rather than degrees: top dead center of the iris is 12 o'clock or 0 minutes, opposite is 6 o'clock or 30 minutes.

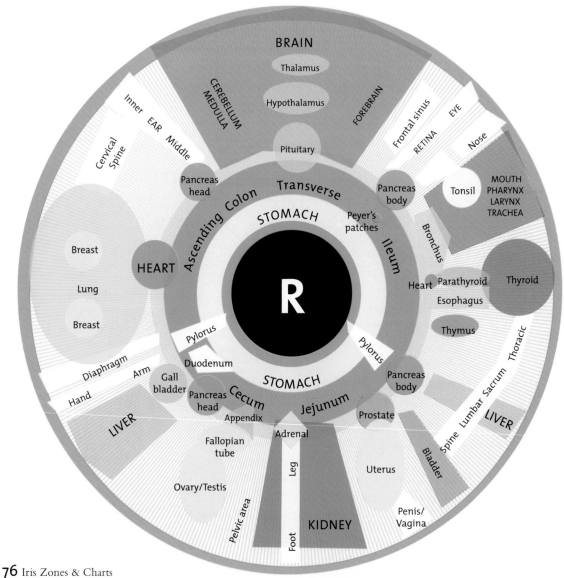

THE BRAIN

Located at 55 minutes and 05 minutes in the left and right irides, the brain contains several reflex areas in the different parts. Note the position of the pituitary gland, and above it, the hypothalamus and the thalamus.

We have already discussed the master hormone gland, the pituitary, on page 48. The hypothalamus, linked to the pituitary below and the thalamus above, controls body temperature, hunger and thirst, sleep, balance, sexual function, and emotional function. It also has links to both the hormonal and autonomic nervous systems through its control of pituitary secretions.

The thalami (there is one in each hemisphere of the brain) are thought to be the seats of conscious awareness of physical stimuli and act as relay stations to transmit these to the lower centers. They also feed into the hypothalamus, hence, sensations received by the thalamus closely affect the functions of this center and also of the pituitary.

The link between mind and body is close to the heart of holistic iridology, and the observation of these items on the chart can give clues as to how susceptible a person may be to stress-related illness. This is amplified if the point diametrically opposite the pituitary, that is at 30 minutes, is also marked. This is usually called the pituitary/adrenal axis. When marked with lacunae, crypts, indentations of the collarette, or radial furrows, it indicates a person who is very sensitive to stress, and who may tend to experience health problems as a result, particularly depletion and exhaustion. However, a lacuna at 0 minutes also can reflect opportunities for developing spiritual insight or psychic abilities. This is the zone that relates to our connection with higher regions of consciousness.

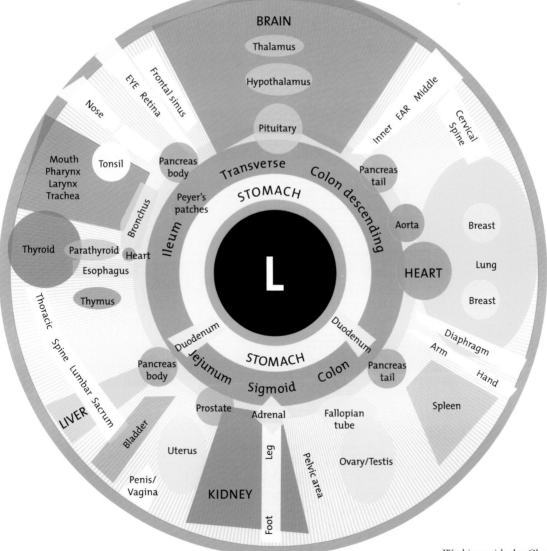

You are now familiar with the arrangement of the gastrointestinal tract around the pupil. You will see that there are some specific areas relating to different parts of the stomach, duodenum, jejunum, small intestine, and ascending, transverse, and descending sections of the colon. Regarding the latter, you can trace the ascending colon from the right eye, the transverse from the right to left eye, and the descending colon down through the left eye, reflecting the peristaltic flow in the colon.

Note the junction of the thin slice describing the esophagus at 45 minutes in the left eye and 15 minutes in the right, with the central ring of the nutritive zone. At this point, a weakness marking could indicate the possibility of a hiatus hernia, as mentioned on page 73. Note also the Peyer's Patches, at about 12 minutes in the right iris and 48 minutes in the left, sitting at the beginning of the small intestine in the intestinal ring. These are a lymphoid aggregation and are a part of our intestinal immune response, as is the appendix (right iris at 32 minutes).

Besides the digestive tract, some other organs need to be assessed as part of the digestive system. These are the liver, gallbladder, and pancreas.

THE LIVER, GALL BLADDER AND SPLEEN

The liver is located in the right iris at 37 to 40 minutes and 22 minutes, and in the left iris at 37 minutes. The gallbladder is at 40 minutes in the right iris, close to the collarette. The spleen is located in the left iris at 20–22 minutes.

The sectors at approximately 20 and 40 minutes in each eye are the liver and spleen reflexes. The liver, being a very large organ, accounts for three of these sites. The liver is situated mainly on the right side of the body. However, the left lobe crosses the median line.

It is very important to assess these areas. The liver does an immense amount of work and can become congested and inflamed. When treated correctly, it regenerates extremely well, so it pays to cleanse and tone it and its many functions from time to time (see page 115 for instructions on how to make the liver-flush drink).

We have already noted that some pigments are hepatotropic, that is, they indicate liver involvement. If they are "topolabile," the influence of the liver extends to the whole body, and signs of its malfunction may be seen in areas other than the specific reflex signs highlighted. However, always check the liver reflexes on the chart. Signs of deficiency—lacunae or rarefaction—may indicate under-functioning, and this can have repercussions on digestion, detoxification, and hormone function. White signs and pigment signs may reveal inflammatory and congestive tendencies.

Likewise, in the spleen, immunity may be weakened if there are signs of deficiency. White irritation signs can signify immune reactivity or allergy, and pigments may imply suppression of immune capability.

Emotional responses

A person's response toward anger, resentment, and frustration also may be revealed here. The liver is the seat of many emotions, and imbalances in its function often will be tied in with failure to process these emotions effectively. Sometimes work on the liver will result in a welling up of such feelings, but this is a transitory reaction. The ability to mobilize emotions and release them is an important part of the way we assert ourselves in life. Persistent or stored anger (resentment) is linked to congestion of the liver, suggested by yellow and brown pigment, or by transversals, and should be regarded as a target for treatment, both physical and psychological. A denial of anger may be linked with insufficiency of the liver, seen in lacunae or rarefaction.

THE PANCREAS

Like the liver, the function of the pancreas has far-reaching effects upon the whole system, yet few people even know where it is and what it does. It is set on the left side of the upper abdomen, behind the stomach. It secretes pancreatic juices, rich in enzymes, which break down food, particularly proteins and carbohydrates.

On the iris chart, the pancreas is situated at approximately 10, 20, 40, and 50 minutes, close to the collarette in both irides. It has eight reflex sites, four in each iris. The position in the left eye

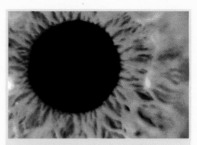

PANCREATIC LACUNA This often can indicate a family history of type II diabetes.

at 20 minutes is the pancreas tail, and this is the most important site to observe to check for a predisposition to type II diabetes (this is where the insulin-producing beta cells in the Islets of Langerhans are mainly situated). A lacuna here frequently shows a family history of diabetes.

The body and the head of the pancreas (left 40 minutes, right 20 minutes and 40 minutes) are more concerned with the provision of digestive juices and enzymes. The sites in the upper portion of the irides (left and right 10 minutes and 50 minutes) are considered to be secondary sites, and do not appear on some charts. However, it has been suggested that these reflect the posterior portion of the organ. Where the collarette is "squared,"

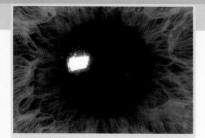

SQUARED COLLARETTE This points to the pancreas, especially its endocrine function for the regulation of blood sugar.

THE HEART

Situated in both irides at 15 minutes and 45 minutes, close to the collarette, the heart is seen in several reflex areas. The position of the heart in the throat area (right iris 15 minutes and left iris 45 minutes) reflects the embryological development of the organ, which takes place in what later becomes the throat. The major reflex site is in the left iris at 15 minutes, as the heart is mainly situated to the left of the body. But because it is close to the center of the body, we also see it reflected in the right iris at 45 minutes.

Lacunae in the heart zone are found frequently, perhaps reflecting the fact that heart disease is still the biggest killer in our society. However, evidence of familial history of heart disease should not be regarded as a death sentence. It is a warning sign telling you to take care of your heart.

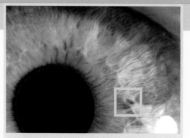

CRYPT IN THE HEART ZONE Widespread throughout the population, these indicate heart problems, possibly heart disease.

A crypt or lacuna in the heart zone may be a sign that you need to embrace life joyfully, and put your worries and anxieties to one side. Many heart attacks occur because people become isolated in their own worlds of worry and stress. To counteract this, it is necessary to relieve the pressure on the heart emotionally as well as physically.

it points to the endocrine function in controlling blood sugar. Bright orange pigments in the iris in any position are amplifying signs. Some researchers have suggested that leaf lacunae appearing anywhere in the region between 20 and 40 minutes in the humoral zone (just outside the collarette) may be interpreted as having pancreatic significance.

Hormonal control

The pancreas secretes the hormones insulin and glucagon, which help regulate blood sugar. Where there are markings in the pancreas reflex sites, especially the pancreas tail in the left eye at 20 minutes, this pattern has been associated with excessive consumption of and craving for sugar or carbohydrates, usually refined, which can lead to an inability to process this sugar, or diabetes mellitus. The pancreas can become exhausted by the demands of a high-sugar diet and fail to secrete adequate levels of insulin.

Lacunae in the endocrine organ reflex sites often indicate that the organ responds over-enthusiastically in the early part of life to become exhausted in later years. The same may be seen in the adrenal glands (30 minutes left and right, at the collarette). There will be a tendency to expend energy immoderately, resulting in fatigue and exhaustion, temporary at first, but possibly eventually chronic.

Note also the positions of other endocrine organs: the testes/ovaries, right 35, left 25 minutes; the pituitary, 0 minutes right and left; and the thyroid, right 13–15, left 45–47 minutes, spanning zones 4 to 6.

THE KIDNEYS

Situated in the right iris at 28 to 31 minutes, and in the left iris at 29 to 32 minutes, the position of the kidneys on the chart may seem strange, being next to the leg in the lower portion of the iris. The kidneys in the body are much higher up, in the mid-back area. However, their chart position reflects their embryological development.

The kidneys are very important to assess due to their role in filtering the

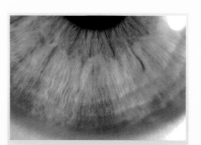

KIDNEY SECTOR RAREFACTION may show a tendency to exhaustion. Other signs highlighting the kidneys are white, cloudy plaques.

blood and removing wastes. Alongside kidney function we also need to assess the skin. If there is a scurf rim, the kidneys are probably doing extra work, and if they show signs of strain then this needs to be addressed.

Lacunae or rarefaction in the kidney zones also can show a tendency to depletion and exhaustion, which can lead to serious consequences, such as chronic fatigue. Topolabile signs that suggest a need to pay attention to the kidneys are white cloudy plaques signifying hyperacidity, and diffuse or straw yellow pigment.

Note also that the reflex area to the leg runs through the kidney zone at 30 minutes. If you see a sign along that line you need to determine which part of the body is involved. A crypt at 30 minutes halfway out to the iris edge can alert you to either a family or individual history of kidney stones.

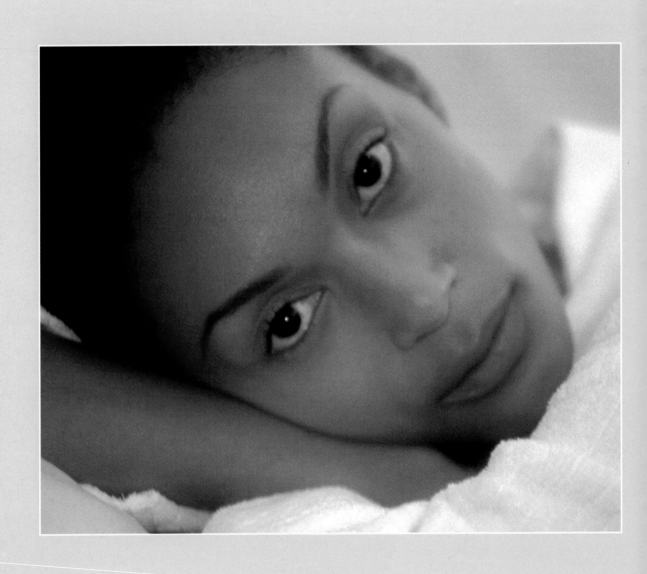

7

ASSESSING YOUR IRIS

By now you may have examined your eyes and discovered some signs, compared them with the iris chart, and perhaps started to think, "Help! I'm falling apart!" Bear in mind that a sign does not indicate a disease, and that most of the signs that you might see in your irides will never become physical problems. Signs should not be interpreted literally without reference to your symptoms, lifestyle, and medical history, and your family, or ancestral medical history. To avoid over-diagnosis, you need to learn how to assess the importance of the signs observed, and how to place them in the context of your life.

An iridology assessment also can direct you to other tests and exploratory procedures that may shed light on your situation. In addition, because iridology concentrates on the causal factors in producing illness, it can help you determine how to reverse the disease process and begin the journey back to health. Even in cases of known degenerative illness, iridology can suggest ways in which health may be safely improved. I've included some standard checklists that will help you to make sense of what you see and make a balanced assessment, as opposed to interpreting signs according to illnesses that they suggest. The first items to consider are symptoms, case history, and iris display.

MAKING A HEALTH ASSESSMENT

Usually, we visit a doctor or health professional because we are experiencing symptoms and, having described these symptoms, the practitioner uses them to form his or her initial assessment of the problem. This is called differential diagnosis and it is the process of determining what the problem is most likely to be by reference to outward signs. The advantage of this approach is the recognition that a pain in, for example, your left arm, may not mean you have a problem with your arm, but that the pain may be due to angina, a serious and potentially life-threatening heart problem. Differential diagnosis is a medical skill that needs to be learned in an appropriate training context. However, symptoms also are likely to be the most common starting point in a self-evaluation, and must be taken into account. Your symptoms are

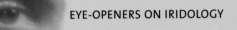

EYE-OPENERS ON IRIDOLOGY

HOLISTIC DIAGNOSIS The meaning of an iris sign may not always be entirely physical. Emotional or psychological concerns may be at the root. Try to treat the whole picture or else you could well overlook important causal factors, and your condition, even if it initially responds to therapy, may well recur.

your body's primary means of communicating its inner distress. Always listen and take note, and then try and find out what they mean.

ASSESSING YOUR SYMPTOMS

Divide your body into separate anatomical systems and study each one: skin, muscles, bones, nerves and brain, hormones, digestion, kidneys and urinary tract, respiratory tract, immune system, heart and circulation, and reproductive organs.

Write down each system as a separate heading and then make a note of whatever you notice about each category, including positive factors as well as negative ones.

CREATING A CASE HISTORY

After listing your symptoms, take down your case history. This can be created at any time but set aside sufficient time for it, as it is important to

In your self-evaluation, list your symptoms and any important details about your habits, previous illnesses, family medical history, medications, etc. creating a thorough survey.

ANATOMICAL SYSTEMS OF THE BODY

System	Organs/parts of body involved	Function
Integumentary	Skin, hair, nails	Protection, regulation of heat, excretion
Lymphatic	Lymph vessels and channels, spleen lymph nodes, lymphoid aggregations (e.g. tonsils, appendix), lymphatic fluid, lymphocytes	Recycling and cleansing of body-fluids, immunity
Musculo-skeletal	Muscles, tendons, ligaments, bones	Movement, protection, stabilization of posture, generation of heat
Cardiovascular	Heart, arteries, veins, capillaries, blood—red and white corpuscles, spleen, lungs	Oxygenation and nourishment of tissues, maintenance of blood pressure
Digestive	Mouth, teeth, esophagus, stomach, small and large intestines, bowel, liver, gallbladder, pancreas, digestive secretions	Assimilation of nutrients, production of energy
Respiratory	Mouth, ears, nose, larynx, pharynx, trachea bronchi, lungs, heart	Oxygenation, excretion
Reproductive—Female	Uterus, fallopian tubes, ovaries, vagina, breasts	Procreation, sexuality
Reproductive—Male	Penis, testes, prostate	Procreation, sexuality
Hormonal (endocrine)	Pituitary, thyroid, parathyroid, pancreas, adrenals, gonads, other organs also having hormone receptors	Communication, regulation, metabolism
Nervous	Brain, spinal column, nerves, eyes	Communication, sensation, movement, thought, and feeling
Immune	Lymph, leucocytes, phagocytes, lymphoid aggregations (tonsils, adenoids), other organs having receptors: pervasive system	Protection and defense against pathogens, tumor surveillance, inflammatory capacity
Urinary	Kidneys, uretors, bladder, urethra, penis	Excretion of waste products, temperature regulation

create a thorough and comprehensive survey of your lifestyle, medical history, and family patterns. Make notes in the categories listed on page 83.

Factors relevant to a case history

- Personal medical history from childhood, including vaccinations, hospitalizations, surgery, medication (including current), etc.
- Family medical history back to grandparents: what illnesses did they suffer; if they have died, how old were they and what did they die of
- If you have children, their medical histories
- Your diet: draw up a chart detailing what you usually have daily for breakfast, lunch, and dinner, and any snacks or drinks, etc. Pay particular attention to how often and how much you eat of potential problem-causing foods, such as dairy products, wheat, and yeast (the most common food allergens). Note any lack of fluid intake (especially water), and the amount of tea and coffee drunk. Also note down your consumption of animal proteins (list what kinds of meat are eaten, and if organically farmed)
- Past dietary patterns or habits
- Other habits, e.g. smoking, alcohol intake, and use of recreational drugs
- Any dietary supplements taken: herbs, homeopathic medicines, vitamins, minerals, etc.
- Frequency of bowel movements
- Any previous experience of alternative or complementary medicine, including homeopathy, acupuncture, osteopathy, or herbalism
- Your job and work history; list any work-related stresses that you experience now or in the past
- Personal relationships: current and previous stresses relating to family and friends and past emotional trauma or bereavements
- Your emotional and mental life: level of satisfaction in life, hobbies, or other pursuits. Do you balance your work, rest, and play?
- Any spiritual beliefs or experiences you have or have had

IRIS DISPLAY

Having made your inventory of symptoms and personal history, you are ready to assess your iris display. Start with the basic constitution associated with your irides: blue, brown-eyed, or mixed. Then assess the structure of your irides (see pages 39–51), and list the four or five signs that stand out to you, and their meanings, for example, lacunae or crypts, pigments, contraction furrows, a scurf rim, or bright white signs. You may find that certain patterns or themes begin to appear. Don't tackle more than four or five signs at first, and choose obvious ones. You also need to assess your energy, stamina, and any other, possibly underlying, influences that may be potential threats.

THE SQUINT TEST

This is a simple way of determining which iris signs are important. You need to squint as you look, blurring your vision. You will immediately lose the details and be left with the most obvious features. The guidelines below will help you choose ones that need further exploration.

1 A sign stands out, e.g. a large lacuna, a big black pigment, or an orange central heterochromia against a blue/gray background. If something is immediately noticeable, look into it.

2 Several signs point to the same organ or system, e.g. small signs in the liver reflex site, yellow or brown pigmentation (topolabile) in other sectors, and pupil flattening adjacent to the liver sector. In this case, whatever the symptoms, you will probably need to treat your liver.

3 Contrasting signs appear in the same organ sector, e.g. bright signs combined with dark signs, such as a deep lacuna bordered by bright white fibers. This shows an area where there may be some conflict, with possibly painful consequences. The bright sign denotes high reactivity, and the dark sign tells you that there is a core of negativity and possible degeneration. The likelihood of symptoms arising in such an area is high.

Also note appearances that suggest problems that may be latent or undiscovered, such as a lipemic or cholesterol ring, which can point to a potentially life-threatening blood condition. Anchor your observations to what is verifiable; for example, if you see a lipemic ring, you can consider taking a cholesterol test, but bear in mind that it may still display a predisposition to a condition rather than a hard-and-fast diagnosis.

You also can start to make deductions from your symptoms and case history about the presence of signs. For example, if you suffered from childhood eczema and have rough irritable skin as an adult, you will want to check to see if you have a scurf rim circling your iris. If you do, you can further deduce that you are having difficulty eliminating toxins and waste products, and you can examine other organs and systems concerned with elimination. From this assessment, you can begin to identify possible causes for the problems you are experiencing. The following guidelines will help you make a quick assessment without looking at specific signs and will also help you to assess your inherent resources.

Color, Structure, and Overlay

See chapter four for color and structural types (for example, the blue iris type and the high resistance type) and chapter five for types of overlay (for example, the lipemic overlay). These suggest possible regulatory disorders and may result in accumulations of acids and other toxins, a buildup of cholesterol, and lymphatic congestion.

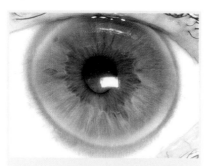

CIRCULARITY DEVIATION
If your iris is not perfectly round, the problems you are experiencing may be due to your nervous system.

Circularity

Observing the circular structures of the irides—the pupillary ruff or pupil margin, the collarette, contraction furrows, and the circularity of the iris—gives you information about your nervous system. Occasionally, the iris is not completely circular, and this may mean that the nervous system is a factor in any problems you are experiencing. Sometimes the disturbance in circularity is obvious. In the picture on the left, there is a flattening of the iris in the lower segment. This person was suffering from extreme pain as a result of rigidity of the lumbar spine, which was relieved by means of osteopathic adjustment. However, there remained a tendency for the same pattern to recur under stress.

Nerve supply problems to the organs may also be important factors to assess, and are suggested by a flattening of the pupil, as well as by indentations or jaggedness of the collarette.

Density

The overall density of iris fiber structure is covered under structural types in chapter four (see page 40). Density is a measure of resistance. In general, the denser your iris, the more resistant you are, and the less dense, the less resistant you are. It is important to know your level of resistance in order to make appropriate adjustments to your lifestyle as part of any treatment. Also, in assessing the impact of stress, your degree of tolerance must be taken into consideration. Your lifestyle may be putting undue strain on your constitution if it is delicate. The measure of

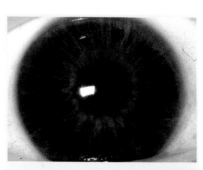

DARK IRIS This may show that your system cannot react sufficiently to protect itself against harmful influences and illnesses.

resistance in individual organs is also important. Note signs of reduced fiber density that may alert you to specific organ problems (see page 57). Low resistance in any area may be seen in features such as lacunae and rarefaction, or a loosening of the texture of the iris.

Shading

This refers to dark or light appearances in the iris, which give information about the ability of your system or of an individual organ to react. Whiteness or brightness shows high reactivity, with a tendency to inflammation; dark and black areas suggest an absence of reactivity, with the danger of failure to act in defense against illnesses and harmful influences, resulting over time in potential tissue degeneration and destruction. A dark iris shows a system that may not be able to react sufficiently to protect itself. A bright, pale iris with whiteness may tend toward over-reactivity and chronic inflammation—the rheumatic iris type.

Assessing individual organs for their ability to react or not, and whether there is a tendency to chronic over- or under-reactivity, can be important. For example, if your iris has a loose texture and dark shading in the kidney sector and you have skin problems, one factor in your condition may be under-functioning of the kidneys, which is a clue to resolving the problem.

ASSESSING FAMILIAL TRAITS

If, when assessing significant signs, you come across something that seems to be important, yet which is not in your case history, it may suggest familial traits. Consider whether anyone in your family has suffered with the problem indicated. Check whether there is any arthritis, high blood pressure, diabetes, heart weakness, or bowel problems in

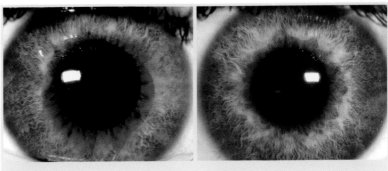

Right eye   Left eye

PATERNAL INFLUENCE The right iris relates mainly to the father's genetic contribution. This boy's right iris is the dominant one (it has the most outstanding signs) so the paternal genes are most influential.

your family. In many cases, health problems experienced by your parents or grandparents may be lying in wait for you as you grow older, and conditions such as breast cancer clearly run genetically through the female line of a family. You also need to assess how likely it is that a problem that seems to be indicated in your iris will actually occur. It is possible that a sign may reflect a family condition that has not surfaced for generations.

How important are these traits when assessing your own health risks or predispositions? If your mother had high blood pressure does that mean you will have the same problem? Bearing in mind that different traits come through different lines of the family, can we predict the inherited elements that we may manifest? The two distinct strands that make up your inheritance are visible in your irides; the right iris relates chiefly to paternal inheritance, the left to maternal. The iris with the most prominent structural signs is the dominant iris. If structure is not conclusive, look at pigment.

In the pictures above we see the irides of a young boy whose dominant genetic influence is paternal. Your eyes may not show such an extreme variation, but if you can determine which iris is dominant, it is a clue as to which of your parents has passed your main health predispositions down to you, and what health threats may most affect you.

SUMMARY OF IRIS ANALYSIS

1 Note any current symptoms.

2 Record your case history.

3 Observe your iris display, noting the following information:
Color—three basic types
Structure/texture—four basic types
Circularity, density, and shading
Note three to five signs that either pervade (e.g. cholesterol ring, hyperacidic clouding) or that stand out in the iris (e.g. a large lacuna, pigment spot, or central heterochromia).

4 Perform a basic crosscheck between symptoms (past and present) and iris indications.

5 If the crosscheck is negative, consider the possible contribution of vital organs—such as the liver and kidneys—to your symptoms (see box on page 84).

6 Consider how your iris display may reflect your family history, where known. If necessary, assess which iris is dominant, that is, the probability of characteristics being passed down from one parent.

7 Construct a three- or four-point health plan that covers your basic indications and helps to prevent the main risks to your health, using the suggestions in chapters three to five.
For example, if you have a lymphatic constitution and a high resistance structure with a hyperacidic overlay, you will need to pay attention to elimination, detoxification, and immunity. You will also need to consider what you can do to balance and nourish your nervous system and pay specific attention to eliminating acids from your body. You also can adopt a diet that will help to minimize acid formation.
If you have a hematogenic constitution, self-protective structure, and lipemic overlay, blood cleansing will be important to keep your blood composition healthy; cayenne and ginger will help to stimulate your circulation; nerve treatments and muscle relaxants will treat your tendency for cramping and nervous tension; and treating your liver will assist in bringing blood fats down to normal levels. In addition, you need to make efforts to clear accumulated fats out of the circulatory vessels.

Drawing a Blank

What do you do if your assessment doesn't make sense, when you see signs that indicate problems that you don't seem to have, when nothing seems to match up, and you do not recognize yourself in your assessment? There are a few reasons why this might happen:

1 The indications are latent tendencies and have not yet manifested. When a problem is likely to appear is different for each person.

2 A symptom is a warning that your constitutional tolerances have been breached. If you live in a way that supports your weak points and avoids threats, the symptom may not appear. Severe problems in the past may be clearly reflected in your iris display, even though you are now free from discomfort through having made the necessary adjustments.

3 You are not ready to become conscious of yourself in this way or you may not want to face the problems. High-resistance type people sometimes find it hard to admit that there may be good cause to change their lifestyles, and they also seem to be able to absorb a lot of stress.

4 You are seeing factors that influence the general environment of the body. We do not generally feel liver congestion, yet when it is a factor, other things may start to malfunction. This is the less immediately verifiable aspect of iridology that works with the concept of the pre-pathological—the slight disturbances of homeostasis or metabolic function that may eventually add up to something more serious. In this case, there is work to be done on a preventive level (see pages 107-117 on cleansing and detoxifying).

5 The indications are emotionally or psychologically significant. If you wish to explore these levels, you will need to seek professional guidance.

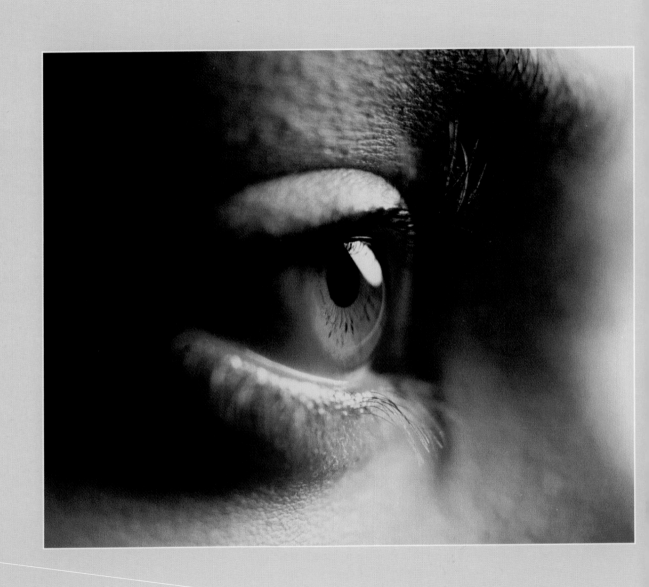

8

COMMON CONDITIONS
SEEN IN THE IRIS

An iris portrait is a collection of indications that point to a particular problem. It is not a hard-and-fast diagnosis; it simply means that there is a high chance of the suggested health problem manifesting. Iris indications also indicate abnormalities or system failures, which over a period of time may bring about a certain condition. By the time you have an identifiable disease, there have usually been many years of pre- or sub-clinical events. Bear in mind that the limits of tolerance in your system, the requirements of homeostasis, are quite narrow. Homeostasis may be described as the process by which the internal systems of the body—pressure, temperature etc.— are maintained in equilibrium, despite variations in external conditions.

The following illustrations are examples of what kinds of appearances suggest possible problems. The principles are energetic—we look to see if an organ is over- or under-active; or showing deficiency or excess. Remember that white equals over-reactive, dark equals under-reactive; loose equals low resistance, tight equals high resistance; lacunae equals emptiness and deficiency; pigment equals fullness and excess.

Arthritis and Rheumatism

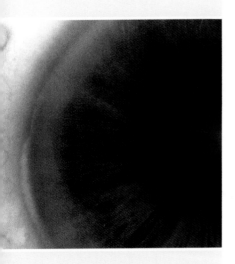

Arthritis and rheumatism are examples of chronic inflammation. They show an ongoing attempt by your body to isolate and resolve a long-standing problem. Where there is inflammation, the tissues are attempting to resolve disruption and repair damage.

There are over 70 different types of arthritis; however, the main types are osteoarthritis and rheumatoid arthritis. The latter is considered to have an autoimmune component (the immune system attacks the body), while the former, far more common form, is most often described as "wear and tear" and 80 per cent of people over the age of 50 have signs of it.

Iris signs do not really distinguish different types of arthritis. While it is sometimes possible to point to a predisposition to arthritis, it is not usually possible to say which kind. However, the rheumatoid variety is more common in people with very pale irides, displaying rheumatic and hyperacidic signs and a tendency to immune-related disorders, while osteoarthritis is found in people with all iris types.

Iris signs

Iris appearances suggesting a predisposition to arthritis and rheumatism:
- A frosted arc known as a spondalarthritic arc (see photo left).
- A rheumatic constitution: a pale lymphatic (blue-eyed) type person, with general whitening of the fibers.
- White or pale yellow cloudy plaques or wisps in the ciliary zone suggesting high levels of uric acid in the tissues. The yellow tinge may indicate impaired kidney function and a toxic bowel.
- General cloudiness of the ciliary zone, suggesting poor resolution of acid wastes, in brown eyes, particularly of the mixed type.
- Transversals criss-crossing in the 4th minor zone (musculo-skeletal zone).
- Signs for rigidity or misalignment of the spinal system, such as pupil flatness, or disturbed circularity of the iris.

In the photo on page 92 of a blue iris we see white cloudy plaques, especially in the 4th minor concentric zone, which reflects the musculo-skeletal system. This describes reactivity and inflammation from high levels of acidic waste. The outer ring of the iris is dark—referred to as a scurf rim—indicating poor skin function and elimination. The flatness of the lumbar reflex at the pupil border is emphasized by a deepening of the scurf rim at that point. The dark color inside the central ring, the intestinal zone, suggests sluggishness of the bowel and retention of toxic wastes,

SUGGESTED REMEDIES

 THERAPIES Bowel cleanse, kidney and liver flush, hydrotherapy

 HERBS Teas or tinctures: ginger, celery seed (anti-inflammatory); black cohosh, wild yam (antispasmodic); yarrow, nettle, cleavers, bogbean, prickly ash, devil's claw (anti-inflammatory and detoxifying). Wild lettuce, valerian, Jamaican dogwood, and black cohosh reduce pain.

A CASE OF ... Arthritis

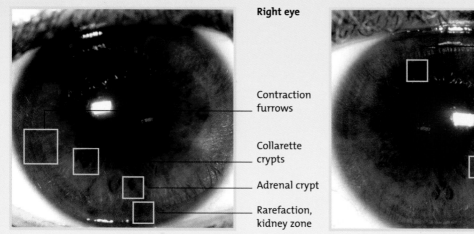

Right eye

Contraction furrows

Collarette crypts

Adrenal crypt

Rarefaction, kidney zone

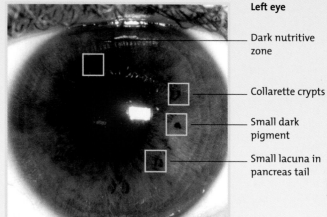

Left eye

Dark nutritive zone

Collarette crypts

Small dark pigment

Small lacuna in pancreas tail

Joanne was 36 years old and had a diagnosis of psoriatic arthritis with symptoms of lupus. Both these conditions are chronic inflammatory connective tissue complaints with an autoimmune element.

Arthritis had come on quickly with little warning. Her doctor wanted to give her immunosuppressive drugs and she had been given a steroid to help control the inflammation, together with a thrice-daily dose of aspirin, none of which she wanted to take long-term.

Joanne suffered from poor circulation and chilblains, felt tired and listless, suffered occasional irritable bowel symptoms, and did not sleep well. Her immunity generally was low, and she caught lots of viral infections.

Although a vegetarian, Joanne relied heavily on sugar, refined carbohydrate products, French fries, and dairy products. She drank more than eight cups of tea or coffee daily (with two teaspoons of sugar), and craved acidic foods such as tomatoes and vinegar—all contraindicated in her condition—and chocolate, especially at the time of menstruation. She did no exercise.

Irides

Her color type is dark mixed, showing a typical pattern of a darker nutritive zone and collarette, and a ciliary zone with lighter, greenish patches. The small dark pigment at 3 o'clock in the left eye, together with the crypts around the collarette, imply autointoxication and a weakening of the immune system. The iris structure is glandular-emotional, with lacunae and crypts around the collarette, particularly in the pancreas and adrenal positions. There are markings in the thyroid zones in both eyes.

There is a lacuna at 4 o'clock in the left eye, close to the collarette, showing a blood sugar problem. Her addiction to sugar supports this, as does squaring of the collarette, especially in the left eye. There was type II diabetes on her mother's side of the family.

Crypts in the adrenal zones in both eyes, with enlarged pupils, suggest adrenal over-activity and exhaustion. Contraction furrows also support this, and the prominent, ropy appearance of the collarette along some of the colon reflex (see the left iris from 55 to 12 minutes and from 18 to 21 minutes) suggests nervous irritability of the bowel that may show an imbalance of the autonomic nerve system, as well as food allergies.

The kidney zones in both eyes show a looser texture and a slightly darker color. There is lightening of the fibers in the left iris at about 20 minutes in the spleen zone, and a breaking of the contraction furrows at that point suggests stress upon immune function.

Treatment

Joanne reformed her diet radically, eliminating tea, coffee, sugar, and the saturated and highly heated fats in the dairy products and fried foods. This relieved pressure on her liver and pancreas. She also cut out acidic foods such as tomatoes, potatoes, peppers, and eggplant, which are common irritants for rheumatism and arthritis.

She ate more fresh, raw fruits and vegetables, drank plenty of filtered water, and took a herbal formula including blood purifiers, digestive bitters, and antispasmodic and nerve-relaxing agents. She also paid attention to her stress levels and became aware of when her body warned that she was exceeding her limits of tolerance through joint pains and skin outbreaks.

Three weeks after her first visit the improvements were dramatic. She still suffered from some symptoms from time to time, especially under stress, but she knew what triggered her condition and how to make changes where necessary.

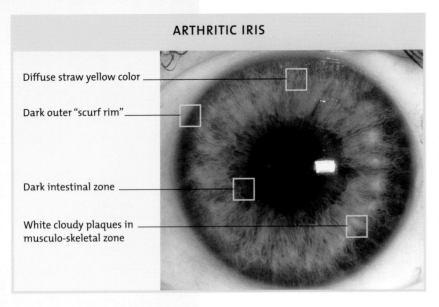

ARTHRITIC IRIS

Diffuse straw yellow color

Dark outer "scurf rim"

Dark intestinal zone

White cloudy plaques in musculo-skeletal zone

which may be reabsorbed by the body, placing stress on the kidneys. The yellow in the upper region shows that kidney function may be impaired, leading to reabsorption of acidic wastes, a potential cause of inflammation. The yellow pigment in the sclera shows disturbance of liver metabolism.

Treatment

Herbal treatments for arthritis include anti-inflammatory and alterative herbs. Alteratives cleanse the blood through acting on the liver, kidneys, and lymphatic system. Sluggishness in the digestive tract also points to poor assimilation of nutrients, and nutrition can help to treat arthritis. Certain foods are contraindicated due to their tendency to create over-acidity or inflammation, and foods that supply minerals, vitamins, trace elements, and micronutrients are required to aid the repair process.

Herbs to use as teas or tinctures include ginger and celery seed (anti-inflammatory); black cohosh and wild yam (antispasmodic); and yarrow, nettle, cleavers, bogbean, prickly ash, and devil's claw (anti-inflammatory and detoxifying). Wild lettuce, valerian, Jamaican dogwood, and black cohosh also may help to reduce pain.

The main focus of treatment for arthritis is to cleanse and detoxify the system, ensuring that all elimination channels are open and active. Assess the bowel, kidneys, liver, and lymph drainage (see pages 113–15).

Apply hydrotherapy locally, ending with hot water in the first stages of treatment (see page 112). After performing this, use a deep heat unguent or embrocation, rubbing it into the affected area to improve circulation and help rebuild tissues. To make your own oil, cover equal parts of ginger root, cayenne berries, St John's wort, arnica, and calendula flowers with olive oil for two weeks, shaking the mixture twice daily. Strain the herbs and add essential oils of peppermint and wintergreen (one drop of essential oil per milliliter). A 50ml bottle contains 25 drops of each oil.

Persevere with exercise to keep your circulation active and your joints supple. Swimming is ideal, as skeletal shock is reduced.

The Gastrointestinal Tract

The iris is a particularly good guide for assessing digestion. Our digestive systems are almost constantly active, and in these days of high-stress living, comfort eating, poor quality food, and other toxic influences and habits, they are under siege. The correct operation of the digestive tract is fundamental to all other organs and systems. Its malfunction is a factor in a range of complaints.

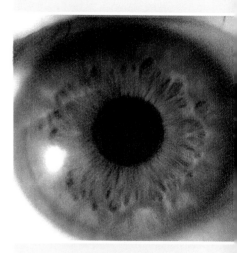

INDIGESTION, ACID STOMACH, AND REFLUX

Excess stomach acidity, indigestion, and esophageal reflux are all suggested by a bright white stomach halo. This implies over-reactivity of the stomach, with an excess production of hydrochloric acid. Reflux occurs when this acid escapes upward into the esophagus, particularly when the valve at the top end of the stomach is weak or damaged. This is known as a hiatus hernia. This weakness can be exacerbated through overeating and eating too many acid-forming foods. Symptoms can appear, which will disappear once eating habits have been corrected.

Iris signs

A hiatus hernia may be shown by a crypt or defect marking at 15 minutes in the right iris, and 45 minutes in the left iris, at the collarette, and at the junction of the reflex to the esophagus and the gastrointestinal tract.

Treatment

Treatment for indigestion, acid stomach, and reflux includes practicing food combining (see page 123), reducing acid-forming foods, and, particularly, reducing your intake of refined wheat products. Use slippery elm powder, marshmallow, and licorice powders in drinks to absorb acids and rejuvenate the stomach lining. Herbs taken as teas or tinctures such as meadowsweet and dandelion normalize stomach secretions, while century herb helps heal a hiatus hernia.

SUGGESTED REMEDIES

 DIET Reduce intake of acid-forming foods and refined wheat products

 HERBS Powders in drinks to absorb acids and repair stomach lining: slippery elm, marshmallow, and licorice; teas or tinctures to normalize stomach secretions: meadowsweet, dandelion; century herb for hiatus hernia.

 THERAPIES Food combining

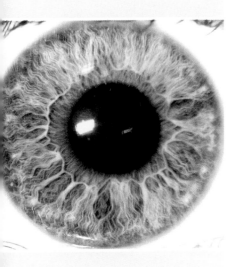

FOOD SENSITIVITY AND IRRITABLE BOWEL SYNDROME

If you have digestive pain or discomfort, the food that you eat is likely to be the cause. The incidence of food allergy or intolerance is high and getting higher. Food sensitivities may be suspected wherever you see brightness and reactivity of the collarette. If you have a hyper-reactive or allergic disposition, there may be reactivity in your gastrointestinal tract, with the accompanying symptoms of griping pain and spasm, alternating constipation and diarrhea, and bloating and distension of the abdomen. This complex of symptoms is often called "irritable bowel syndrome" (IBS), and the nerves and stress are frequently involved.

Food intolerances may cause other symptoms, and cutting out the offending foods may relieve other allergic tendencies such as hay fever and asthma, as well as general fatigue, reduced mental function, and depression. Sensitivity to otherwise healthful foods also might be reduced by a period of recuperation, where you reduce aggravating influences such as stress and unhealthy food, and strengthen and rebuild the digestive system.

Iris signs

Hypersensitivity of the gastrointestinal tract is most often seen in blue-eyed people because of their heightened reactivity. A prominent, ropy, or jagged collarette may indicate this tendency in people of any eye color. Strong coloring of the collarette can add to the diagnosis. In the picture below, note not only the whiteness of the collarette, but also the yellow pigment in the upper and right segments. This indicates involvement of the liver, and a high probability of sensitivity or intolerance to dairy fats.

Treatment

Treatment for food sensitivity and irritable bowel syndrome includes identifying possible allergens, for example dairy foods, wheat, and yeast. Treat your nerves with the following herbs, taken as teas or tinctures: skullcap, passionflower, or valerian. Antispasmodic herbs that can be used include wild yam, black cohosh, and peppermint. Practicing food combining and taking bitter tonics will promote better digestion, thus minimizing potentially aggravating matter entering the colon. Pau d'Arco, barberry root bark, black walnut hulls, and wormwood improve gastrointestinal immunity and control candida. People suffering from these problems should try to reduce their stress levels.

SUGGESTED REMEDIES

 DIET Identify possible allergens, such as dairy foods, wheat, and yeast.

 HERBS For the nerves: teas or tinctures of skullcap, passionflower, valerian; antispasmodic herbs: wild yam, black cohosh, peppermint; for digestion: bitter tonics; for gastrointestinal immunity: Pau d'Arco, barberry root bark, black walnut hulls, wormwood

 THERAPIES Food combining

A CASE OF ... Ulcerative Colitis

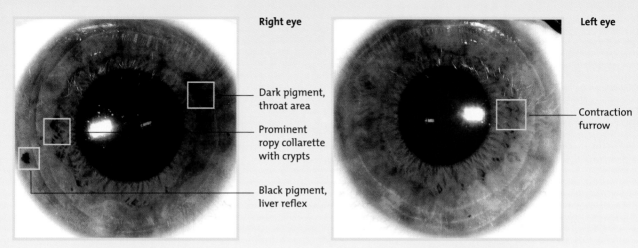

Right eye

Dark pigment, throat area

Prominent ropy collarette with crypts

Black pigment, liver reflex

Left eye

Contraction furrow

Twenty-four-year-old Alice came to me suffering from severe bleeding ulcerative colitis, as a result of which she had been recommended steroids. When she expressed concern about this, her doctor told her that if she did not accept treatment she would probably develop cancer in later life. However, she managed to get a prescription for non-steroidal, anti-inflammatory, antispasmodic drugs.

Her condition was obviously stress-related: her symptoms became worse when work conditions were challenging or uncontrollable. She was also frustrated by her job. She revealed that she had taken her position in order to make a living from a sustainable career but that she really wanted to train as an actor. I pointed out that she owed it to herself to fulfill her potential.

There also were dietary factors. When she was free of symptoms she would adopt bad habits, only to suffer the consequences.

Irides
Her constitution is hematogenic, with a light, cloudy ciliary zone, collarette crypts, and dark "tar" pigments in the right iris. These show a risk of serious immune weakness.

The noticeable structural features are in the digestive reflex area around the pupil, with a looser texture and a prominent, ropy collarette, with many crypts, mainly in the ascending and descending colon reflexes. This implies irritability and sensitivity of the colon, including possible food allergies. Also, in each iris there is a contraction furrow appearing inside the collarette, in the reflex area of the colon, denoting a focus for stress in this area.

The black pigment in the right iris shows potential weakness in her immune system. The dark sector in the right iris between 10 and 20 minutes shows crypts and broken contraction furrows, indicating a focal area for stress and reduced drainage and immunity. Energetically, her issues are connected with self-expression, speaking, and manifesting one's inner truth, as well as grief, and a yearning for reconnection to creative energy.

Alice wanted to be an actor, but, she also had a deep mistrust of this impulse, and a feeling that it was necessary to conform to conventional notions of a respectable career. By overriding her deeper desire, she was suppressing a vital aspect of herself, and causing irritation and resentment to surface as a physical problem.

Bleeding from the bowel symbolically expressed her feeling that she was letting her lifeblood drain away and life pass her by. She was facing an opportunity to make deep changes in her life, even though this might mean challenging family and social pressures. Her personality also had a measure of self-sacrifice, which was draining her, and making it difficult for her to change direction. She was being challenged to put herself first and assert herself in a way that she had perhaps never done before.

Treatment
When Alice was strict with her diet, her condition improved. However, my assessment put priority on psychological considerations, which are often significant in ulcerative colitis.

Avoiding dairy products and wheat/gluten products, eating raw foods and drinking juices, and taking herbal remedies and performing detoxification routines all helped, but at the first sign of stress, the symptoms returned, sometimes with a vengeance. I strongly suspected that she would not obtain relief from her condition until she addressed the underlying frustrations regarding her career.

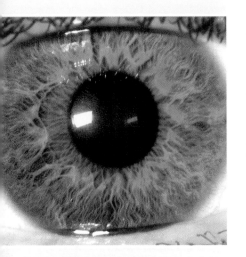

SLUGGISH DIGESTION

People with a mixed iris type often have signs that show a more sluggish digestive system. If there is pigmentation over the digestive zone in the iris, there may be a shortfall in the person's ability to secrete sufficient enzymes for digestion. The result will be discomfort or pain experienced within half an hour of eating, with a feeling of tightness and distension around the midriff. Symptoms may often be worse toward the evening, and eating too late is likely to exacerbate the problem. Pigment also may be present in people with blue or gray eyes, and may indicate a problem with the supply of enzymes for digestion.

Iris signs

Left is a picture of a blue eye with an orange central heterochromia. The individual suffered from severe bloating whenever she ate.

A dark nutritive zone, with perhaps a tinge of brown/gray, also can suggest low energy and sluggishness of digestion. Combined with a thin or invisible collarette, this can show a failure to absorb nutriment, which may result in reduced gastrointestinal immunity, candidiasis, and chronic fatigue.

Treatment

A sluggish digestion can be resolved not only by changes in the individual's diet, but also by drinking herbal tinctures containing bitters, which stimulate the secretion of digestive fluids from the liver, gallbladder, and pancreas. The orange color in this person's iris shows that her problem originated from the pancreas, and so food-combining principles were also part of the recommendations (see page 123). Taking care not to overload the digestive system with unsuitable combinations of foods protects the pancreas and extends its functional life.

SUGGESTED REMEDIES

Sluggish digestion

THERAPIES Food combining

HERBS Tinctures containing bitters.

Spasmodic disorders

HERBS Teas or tinctures of wild yam, black cohosh

Constipation
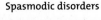
HERBS Atonal constipation: teas or tinctures of senna, cascara, aloe; laxatives: linseeds, psyllium husk, slippery elm powder, licorice powder; spastic colon and colitis: wild yam, black cohosh; bile promotion: gentian, barberry, wormwood, bitter herbs.

SPASMODIC DISORDERS

As we have seen, the nervous system plays a large part in the health of the gastrointestinal tract, and people of the self-protective type (see page 46) are particularly predisposed to gastrointestinal spasms. This can be seen in the radial furrows in the iris, sometimes called "spasm furrows."

Iris signs

Radials show high levels of gastrointestinal stress, and are associated with cramping and spasmodic pain in the gut. Major radials also are seen to cut through the collarette and may weaken the nerve supply for digestion. In the picture (right) the collarette is contracted toward the pupil in a "drawstring" effect, implying poor gastrointestinal dynamics and spasms.

Treatment

Herbs include wild yam and black cohosh, taken as teas or tinctures.

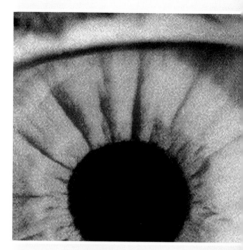

Spasm furrows

CONSTIPATION

There are two basic types of constipation: spastic and atonal, and they need different treatments. It is best to seek professional advice. With spastic constipation, the emphasis is on releasing and relaxation. With atonal constipation (see below right), the peristaltic muscles must be activated.

Constipation also may occur through insufficient secretion of bile from the liver/gallbladder, a lack of hydration, and eating an excess of animal fats and proteins and refined carbohydrates. The ideal frequency of bowel movement is one shortly after each meal.

Iris signs

Spastic constipation (see above right) may appear with a tightly contracted collarette and radial furrows. Atonal constipation appears as distension of the collarette, possibly with lacunae or crypts in the nutritive zone.

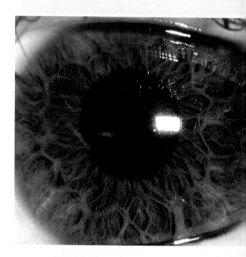

Distended collarette

Treatment

Herbal teas or tinctures to relieve constipation include senna, cascara, and aloe for atonal constipation; linseeds, psyllium husk, slippery elm powder, and licorice powder act as bulking laxatives; wild yam and black cohosh help a spastic colon and colitis, IBS, and diverticulitis; gentian, barberry, wormwood, and bitter herbs promote bile production, a natural laxative.

The Hormone System

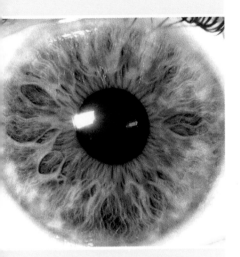

Right eye

The hormone system is one of the body's two important messenger networks, the other being the nervous system. The hormonal organs are all interconnected in a unified system, which is largely controlled by the master gland in the brain, the pituitary, which sends triggering hormones throughout the body to stimulate regulatory activity by the other endocrine glands.

We can see the interdependency of the hormonal organs when someone with very active adrenals—who is always on the go—develops a craving for sweet things. At first, this craving seems to be a symptom of a problem with the pancreas. However, the adrenals cause the person's system to speed up, using up more energy and needing to replace it, and causing other endocrine organs to over-function. In this case, the pancreas secretes more insulin and blood sugar drops, creating a craving for more sugar.

One of the dangers of this scenario is that the individual's system becomes exhausted prematurely. Type II diabetes is often a result of pancreatic burn-out. The tendency to immoderate and uncontrolled output is one of the factors responsible for bringing on the disease. Over-indulgence in refined sugars, carbohydrates, and other glycemic foods speed up the eventual crash.

SUGGESTED REMEDIES

 DIET Reduce intake of refined sugars

 HERBS For digestion: teas or tinctures of gentian, centaury, wormwood, garlic, fenugreek, and neem.
To normalize blood sugar: burdock, Siberian ginseng, bilberry

 THERAPIES Food combining

HYPOGLYCEMIA/DIABETES

Iris signs

A tendency to diabetes/hypoglycemia is indicated by any combination of the following factors:
• A person with the glandular/emotional structural type
• Leaf lacuna or crypt at 4 o'clock in the left iris (pancreas tail)
• Shiny orange pigments anywhere in either iris
• Square shape of the collarette
• Violet hue inside the collarette (nutritive zone)
• Hematogenic constitution
• Lipemic ring (there is a close connection between high blood fats and diabetes)

The pictures above and right show a general hormone imbalance. This 49-year-old man did not have diabetes or a thyroid disorder, although he was clearly hypoglycemic. His symptoms were general debility and fatigue, but his irides revealed that care of the endocrine and digestive systems were probably important in his recovery, and this proved to be the case. His irides show a person with a mixed constitution and a glandular-type disposition. The central heterochromia is orange, and the collarette shows distinct squaring, emphasizing the pancreatic points in both irides.

At 4 o'clock in the left iris we see a leaf lacuna, which is echoed in the right iris by another, larger, one at 8 o'clock, suggesting weakness of the pancreas both hormonally and in terms of digestion.

Other hormonal signs are also evident, notably the thyroid (9 o'clock in the left iris, 3 o'clock in the right), and the adrenals (see the crypt at 32 minutes in the right iris, indentation of the collarette, and an open lacuna at 30 minutes in the left iris). Additionally, observe the small dark crypt at 12 o'clock in the left iris, on the site of the pituitary gland, and another crypt in the region of the hypothalamus, in the right iris at 12 o'clock, further out into the ciliary zone. There are a large number of signs indicating digestive functions.

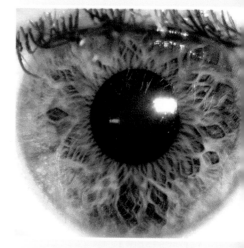

Left eye

Treatment

In order to restore hormonal function, digestion should always be treated alongside any other specific concerns. The most appropriate herbs to use, as teas or tinctures, are bitter herbs, such as gentian, centaury, and wormwood. Garlic, fenugreek, the Indian herb neem, and herbs that normalize blood sugar, such as burdock, Siberian ginseng, and bilberry are also effective. Practicing food combining, see page 123, and reducing your intake of refined sugars, especially sucrose, will also help.

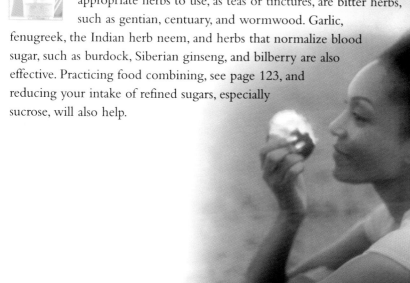

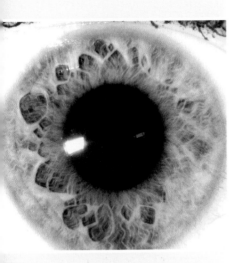

SUGGESTED REMEDIES

 HERBS For the pituitary gland: teas or tinctures of vitex agnus castus, dong quai; estrogenic herbs: red clover, black cohosh, sage; estrogenic foods: soy products, pulses; uterine tonics: partridge berry, raspberry leaf; uterine astringents: lady's mantle, shepherd's purse, cranesbill; to reduce cramping: black cohosh, cramp bark; to relieve PMS: valerian, hops, black cohosh, St John's wort, bearberry (for water retention); for thrush etc.: golden seal, tea tree essence in olive oil

THE FEMALE HORMONE SYSTEM

This system is closely connected with the other endocrine organs. Many women become hypoglycemic at the time of menstruation. Also, women need strong adrenals during the menopause because the ovaries stop producing estrogen and some is produced by the adrenals. Women who avoid excess stress and take adrenal-boosting herbs such as Siberian ginseng, astragalus, and licorice are likely to have an easier menopause.

The appearance of signs in the pituitary and adrenal zones is important when assessing the health of the menstrual cycle. If a woman has menstrual problems, these organs need to be assessed and addressed.

Irides

The picture left shows the right iris of a 21-year-old woman with menstrual cramps, sickness, water retention, and premenstrual tension. Her constitution is lymphatic, her disposition is glandular-emotional, and there is a significant hyperacidic overlay—cloudiness of the ciliary zone.

Among the glandular signs, note the small rhomboid crypt at 12 o'clock at the collarette, a typical pituitary sign, and a larger crypt at around 29 minutes at the site of the adrenal gland. When the pituitary and adrenals are marked, for men or women, there may be a tendency to stress-related disorders. The nausea this woman experienced at menstruation suggested hypoglycemia, and the presence of leaf lacunae, particularly in the lower sector of the iris, indicated pancreatic/prediabetic concerns.

There is an openness and lack of resistance in the lower sector of the iris. This sector contains the kidney, uterus, and ovaries reflexes. It is essential to keep this area well drained and free from toxins, for example, by using castor oil packs, see pages 108–9. The left iris shows distension and loose structure in the sigmoid colon. Anatomically, this part of the colon is curled around the back of the uterus and the ovaries. Any congestion in this part of the colon has an impact on the health of the female organs. Furthermore, at menstruation, when the uterus enlarges, the whole area is put under pressure by any congestion in the colon.

Water retention is suggested by extreme rarefaction in the kidneys, and by the hyperacidic overlay. Pelvic inflammatory disease describes what we see in this picture and it is possible that there is some endometriosis.

Treatment

See the list of herbal remedies in the left-hand column.

A CASE OF ... Endometriosis

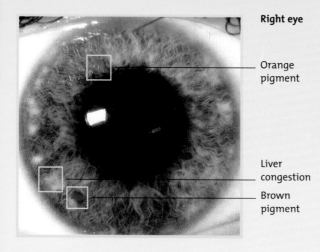

Right eye

— Orange pigment

— Liver congestion

— Brown pigment

Left eye

— Contracted collarette with spasr furrows

— Congestioi spleen

— Darker, loo kidney anc pelvic area

Tricia was 38 years old and had endometriosis, a painful condition in which tissue that forms the inner lining of the uterus grows around the outside of the uterus and in and around the abdominal cavity. It caused painful, heavy periods, mid-cycle pain and bleeding, and nausea and vomiting. She also became very hypoglycemic at menstruation.

She had taken hormone drugs for three years, which had worked quite well, but latterly seemed ineffective or made things worse. A hormone coil had been implanted to suppress menstruation, but it caused pain and was removed.

Other symptoms included swellings and cysts in her neck and breasts (since the hormone treatment), nervous digestion, anxiety, and constipation. A scan revealed uterine fibroids and polyps, and an ovarian cyst.

Her family history included bowel cancer, stroke and circulatory difficulty, osteoarthritis, and anxiety. Her diet was high in carbohydrates and animal proteins and caffeine; she drank very little water; and smoked.

Irides

Her irides are of the lymphatic type (blue), with a lymphatic rosary (white beads around the edge of the iris). There is impaired lymphatic drainage, showing a tendency to lymphatic swellings and cysts. Her lymph system became overloaded as a result of the drugs she was taking.

There are numerous orange and red/brown pigments in the irides, suggesting weakening of the liver (toxicity) and pancreas (blood sugar abnormality and digestive function).

The collarette is contracted toward the pupil margin, and the nutritive zone is narrow, showing poor digestion. At the top, the collarette appears to touch the pupil margin, indicating a spastic colon, constipation, and poor digestion. The collarette has a whitish flare into the upper region of the iris, showing phlegmatic conditions of the gastrointestinal tract. There are small radial furrows in the left iris (also in the upper segment), indicating stress affecting the stomach and possible pre-ulcerative conditions. Both of these signs also suggest toxic headaches and are indicative of high levels of stress.

The lower quadrants in both irides are looser in structure and darker in color, indicating poor drainage via the kidneys, congestive conditions in the pelvic basin, and stress around issues of identity, self-esteem and stamina.

The liver reflex in the right iris (8 o'clock) shows a wedge of white fibers and a thickening of the lymphatic flocculation—a bright white spot in the peripheral zone indicating congestion involving phlegm. There is similar whitening at 4 o'clock in the right iris (liver) and in the left iris (spleen).

Treatment

The priority for lymphatic people is to detoxify, and if there is a rosary in the iris, this is amplified. I activated her bowels, liver, kidneys, skin, and lymphatics. She began a detoxification program including increasing water consumption, performing kidney and liver flushes (see pages 114–15), bowel cleansing (see page 113), dry skin brushing (see pages 110–11), and hydrotherapy (see page 112), paying attention to the lower abdomen using castor oil packs (see pages 108–9). She juiced fresh organic fruits and vegetables, adopted a vegetarian diet, and stopped drinking coffee and smoking. I prescribed herbs to assist her liver, digestion, kidneys, adrenals, lymph system, and hormone system.

Her first menstruation after treatment was much less painful. After six months of treatment she rarely experienced pain as before. Her periods were lighter, and she had no mid-cycle symptoms. A scan revealed that the size of her ovarian cyst had reduced.

Respiratory Disease

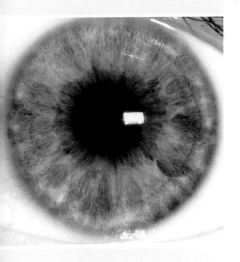

The respiratory system is the body's way of digesting oxygen, and it is vital to keep it in good working order. Giving up smoking is an absolute prerequisite for recovery from respiratory disease.

Iris signs

The most common signs for lung disease are rarefaction and open lacunae, often containing other signs in the sector—transversals, defect markings, tophi (white cotton-wool-like spots showing lymphatic congestion), and contraction furrows, especially if they are broken or interrupted in the lung reflex field. Another sign—a tubercular miasm—also shows a predisposition to lung disease. It may be identified by the following traits:

• Waving or floating fibers that seem to have become detached from the iris, particularly from the collarette, sometimes draping over the pupil
• Wavy "combed hair" appearance of the surface layer of iris fibers
• Lacuna, crypt, or dark rarefaction in the upper right lung reflex area (right iris 45–50 minutes)
• The spondalarthritic arc, (see page 90)

Treatment

People with these signs must focus on immunity, as the implication is that there is an inherited weakness. Their immune systems may be over-reactive.

ASTHMA
Iris signs

Causes for asthma vary between individuals. Some possible scenarios are:

• Allergic asthma: white signs, lymphatic rosary, fine thread-like vessels in the white of the eye and at the limbus or iris edge (allergic tendency)
• Nervous asthma: criss-cross fibers in lung zone ("neuronal net"), contraction furrows, especially where broken in the lung zone (lungs are a focus for stress and psychosomatic disorder)
• Congestive asthma: rarefaction in both lung and kidney zones (insufficient drainage—the lungs may fill up with fluid)

In the photo, note the dark sectors at 3 o'clock and 6 o'clock in the left lung and kidney; white, congestive signs in the 5th minor zone (lymphatics), and contraction furrows breaking in the lung at 3 o'clock.

Treatment

See the list of herbal remedies in the left-hand column.

SUGGESTED REMEDIES

Asthma

 HERBS For nervous asthma: teas or tinctures of anemone, lime tree flowers; for anxiety: lobelia (seek professional advice before use), wood betony, valerian, passionflower; for an allergic component: plantain leaf, echinacea, nettle; to drain excess fluids: dandelion, wild carrot, buchu, golden rod; as a bronchodilator: coffee, ephedra (seek professional advice before use); for sore mucous membranes: marshmallow herb tea

Skin Problems

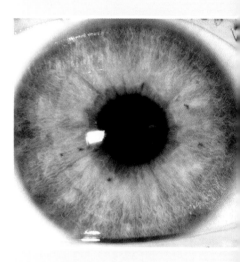

Three general factors influence skin disorders: the nervous system (including emotional issues and stress), filtration and purity of the blood (depending on the liver and kidneys), and the immune system (allergy and autoimmune disturbances).

People who suffer from inflammatory skin problems often notice that their condition worsens under stress. The skin is your boundary with the outer world, and a skin problem may represent a conflict with your environment or close acquaintances. There is sometimes a need to acknowledge irritation, anger, or resentment as part of releasing the condition.

The presence of a scurf rim in the iris nearly always signifies involvement of the skin. It may only be dry or itchy skin or it may be eczema or psoriasis. The scurf rim is also a sign for toxicity due to inefficient elimination. This "holding on" also applies to emotions; there may be difficulty admitting to feelings or holding on to difficult feelings.

Iris signs
The photograph reveals a typical picture suggestive of a disposition to skin problems. The constitution is lymphatic—the rheumatic sub-type (whiteness of fibers), suggesting high reactivity. The iris is dense—a high resistance type, with sensitivity indicated by the contraction furrows. There is a very deep and dark scurf rim.

Brown pigment around the collarette is hepatotropic, reflecting possible disturbances with the liver, and there is a zigzag irritation fiber in the main liver zone at 8 o'clock. It is likely that the liver has been under stress. At the nasal margin of the iris we see many threadlike broken vessels in the sclera (white of the eye), which indicates an allergic tendency.

Treatment
Alterative herbs, or blood purifiers, are effective for conditions such as eczema and psoriasis, working to improve the function of the liver and kidneys. One of my clients, a 49-year-old man, had taken steroids to treat his eczema for so long that his skin was breaking and bleeding every time he banged it or brushed it. If he stopped the steroids, his eczema flared uncontrollably. We stopped the steroids, cleansed the blood, and pacified the nervous system, and his skin began to regain its stability. (See the list of herbal remedies in the right-hand column.)

SUGGESTED REMEDIES

HERBS Teas or tinctures of mountain grape root (*Berberis aquifolium*), burdock root, red clover, echinacea; for the nerves: skullcap passionflower; for eczema and psoriasis: milk thistle (for psoriasis and as a liver tonic), alteratives and blood purifiers

The Kidneys and Urinary Tract

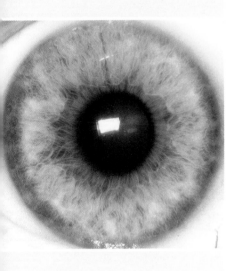

Inadequate kidney function may cause a great many problems, including high blood pressure, skin problems, arthritic and rheumatic disease, asthma, water retention and swelling of the extremities, and other congestive conditions, for example, sinusitis and general lymphatic sluggishness.

You can frequently observe rarefaction, or loosening of the fiber structure, in the kidney zone, and this is an important sign in the assessment of chronic fatigue and debility. There is a close connection between the kidneys and the adrenals. In Chinese medicine, depletion of kidney "chi" (energy) is a noted cause of debility and exhaustion, similar to what Western medicine might refer to as adrenal exhaustion.

The presence of crypts in the kidney zones sometimes shows a tendency to form kidney stones. They also can show that a family member experienced this problem, usually the father. If there is a hyperacidic overlay (cloudy iris), then this tendency is amplified.

Iris signs

The bladder reflex is found in the right iris at 23 minutes and in the left iris at 38 minutes. Whiteness or bright fibers in this sector may reveal a tendency to cystitis. It is also important to look at the smaller reflex sites for the ureters (passages from the kidneys to the bladder) and the urethra (outlet from the bladder).

Treatment

Your water consumption must be adequate; check that you are drinking at least two liters a day. Also, drinking cranberry juice is effective for relieving the symptoms of cystitis. Buchu herb and bearberry, taken as teas or tinctures, act as diuretics and antiseptics; marshmallow root soothes the urinary tract; horsetail and agrimony act as urinary astringents for over-frequent urination and urination at night; and gravel root and hydrangea root are effective for dissolving stones.

SUGGESTED REMEDIES

 DIET At least 2 liters of water a day; cranberry juice for cystitis

 HERBS Teas or tinctures of buchu herb, bearberry as diuretics and antiseptics; for the urinary tract: marshmallow root; urinary astringents: horsetail, agrimony; for dissolving stones: gravel root, hydrangea root

A CASE OF ... Kidney Stones

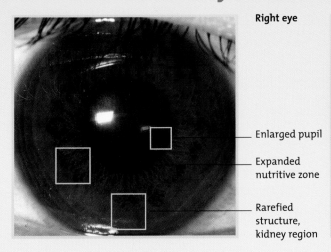

Right eye

- Enlarged pupil
- Expanded nutritive zone
- Rarefied structure, kidney region

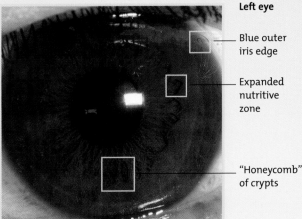

Left eye

- Blue outer iris edge
- Expanded nutritive zone
- "Honeycomb" of crypts

Raju is a 40-year-old Nepalese traditional doctor, or "medicine man." His symptoms were renal colic (pain as a probable result of stones trapped in the narrow passages of the kidneys or ureters) and hematuria (blood in the urine). The likely cause was kidney stones; however, an ultrasound scan was not conclusive. He had suffered the same problem 18 to 20 years ago.

His life was highly stressful because he was the most well-known and sought after practitioner in his tradition, and he was also the last surviving person who could preserve this knowledge. He wanted to set up a foundation for the preservation and dissemination of his tradition. He was working extremely hard and had a lot of stress.

His diet was a strong factor in his symptoms. He drank a glass of water and lemon juice every morning, but then drank no water for the rest of the day. At every house call he was offered millet wine, amounting to more than a bottle a day.

His meals were mainly chicken and vegetables with rice, but were always highly salted, and he drank two glasses of cola daily. He was significantly dehydrated and suffered from constipation, passing bowel motions every other day.

Irides

Raju has a pure hematogenic constitution. His tendency is toward accumulation and excess, and he has a predisposition to toxicity and metabolic disorders of the blood. The formation of stones is typical for people of this type.

The nutritive zone is expanded, with crypts and lacunae in the collarette. This suggests gastric structural tendencies, and reflects a predisposition to digestive sluggishness and constipation. The honeycomb of crypts just inside the collarette in the left eye at about 27 minutes suggests trouble in the sigmoid colon.

There is a blue tinge to the edge of the iris, indicating congestion and stagnation of venous circulation, adding to the impression of congestive conditions of the blood. Contraction furrows and an enlarged pupil (seen particularly in the right iris) attest to internalized stress, but also to an ability for focused activity. The open structure and crypts in the nutritive zone suggest constipation, but also a highly developed instinctual nature and ability to follow gut feelings.

There is localized darkness and rarefaction in the kidney zones—in the right iris at 29 minutes, and in the left at 31 minutes, with crypts—often associated with kidney stones.

Treatment

The priority was to resolve his bleeding. He performed a herbal dissolvent routine daily. This involved juicing apples to produce two liters of juice, then bringing this to the boil with an ounce each of gravel root (*Eupatorium purpurea*) and hydrangea root (*Hydrangea arborescens*). Half an ounce of marshmallow root was added to lubricate and soothe the urinary passages. Raju used a sieve when he urinated to see if he passed deposits.

By the third day of this treatment the bleeding had subsided and he had passed a 3–4 mm stone. He has not had any repeat of the problem, drinks more water, and eats a less salty diet. Activating the bowels and cleansing the blood formed the second stage of treatment, to help prevent a recurrence.

Passing blood possibly symbolized a sense of powerlessness and futility, as well as frustration in his mission to protect and preserve his traditional medical knowledge. He eventually succeeded in setting up a foundation for the preservation of this knowledge, and a school in Nepal in which to teach traditional medicine.

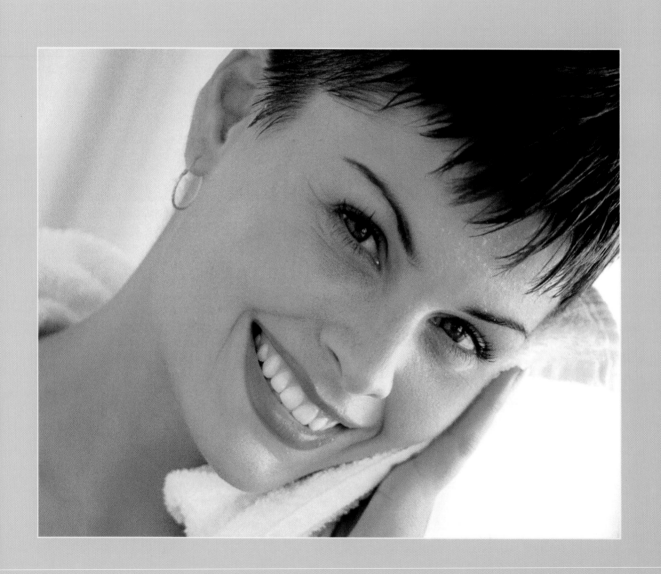

9

DETOXIFICATION ROUTINES

On the following pages, you will find easy detoxification techniques that can be simply and safely performed in your own home yet can be very powerful in both preventive and curative treatments. Most of these routines remove obstructions to health; they detoxify through the eliminative channels of the body and restore healthy functioning to the whole system. They can be used at routine intervals as a preventive measure or as part of a program to restore optimum health after a period of illness.

Your body performs detoxification on a daily basis. However, many of us either exceed "safe" limits of toxic ingestion in our daily diets and through other habits such as drinking alcohol or smoking, or else we may have inherent tendencies to weaknesses in our eliminative processes. These factors may be aggravated by the effects of physical, emotional, and mental stress.

Castor Oil Packs

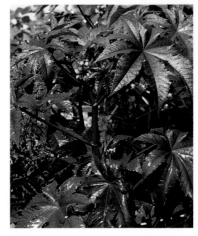

CASTOR OIL PLANT

Castor oil can be used to break up and draw out congestion through the skin. It can be valuable in relieving symptoms of menstrual disorders and to ease the pain of colitis and diverticulitis. It also can be used to decongest the liver and kidneys. In these cases, packs are applied to the abdomen. Packs also can be applied to the neck, under the arm, or in the groin area to relieve lymphatic swellings.

CONDITIONS TO TREAT

The key word for conditions that may benefit from this treatment is congestion. Fluids and waste materials build up where the tissues are unable to drain effectively through the usual channels, and this results in congestion.

Congestive disorders

Iridology is very good at picking out areas that may exhibit signs of pain, inflammation, and swellings—the chief symptoms of congestion. If the bowels, kidneys, liver, or the lymphatic vessels are under-functioning or blocked, they will produce a buildup of waste materials, which then causes inflammation and irritation in the localized area affected.

Pelvic inflammatory disease (PID)

This is a catch-all disorder for a variety of problems affecting women's generative organs, which may include menstrual difficulties, ovarian cysts, fibroids, and endometriosis. Often, abdominal symptoms are found to be a result

How to Prepare and Use a Castor Oil Pack

WHAT YOU WILL NEED

- Good quality castor oil. You can buy this in most supermarkets or health food shops. The best type is organic.
- A piece of soft, undyed, unbleached cotton cloth
- Some plastic wrap or sheeting
- A towel
- A hot water bottle or heat pack

If you have problems such as the ones mentioned above, you should perform this routine every other day or twice a week. Sometimes you may notice that there are yellow or brown deposits on the cloth when you take it off. This indicates that toxins and impurities are being drawn out through the skin. If this happens, throw the cloth away. Otherwise, it can be washed and reused for the next application.

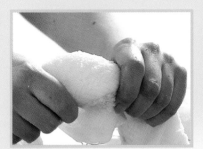

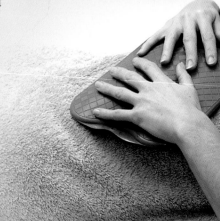

of constipation or an infrequently evacuated bowel. Fecal matter stored in the sigmoid colon, the "S"-bend at the lower end of the colon, begins to leak toxicity into the surrounding tissues. The female reproductive organs are in very close proximity, so they suffer the most from any leakage.

Adhesions

An occasional side effect of gynecological or genitourinary surgery, adhesions are another frequent cause of abdominal pain. Even keyhole surgery can have far-reaching consequences in this regard. Whenever you cut the body, it has to repair itself. In order to do this it secretes a sort of glue, and in order to make sure the job is done properly, it uses plenty of it. This can result in a "sticking together" of internal tissues and organs, known as adhesions. A castor oil pack is considered a specific remedy for adhesions, and will soften, dissolve, and remove the obstruction in a gentle and natural way, yet without "ungluing" the wound itself.

CONTRAINDICATIONS

You should not use a castor oil pack if you are pregnant or breastfeeding. Also, you should not apply one to an open wound.

TAKE CARE

The castor oil plant (*Ricinus communis*) is extremely toxic to humans and animals and if ingested results in death. The toxin contained in castor beans is ricin, a water-soluble protein, which is concentrated in the seed, although the rest of the plant is considered to be slightly toxic as well. Commercially prepared castor oil contains no toxins at all.

1 Warm 4 to 5 tablespoons (50 ml) of castor oil in a pan to a temperature just bearable on the skin.

2 Soak the cloth in the oil for about a minute, then gently squeeze out any excess oil, but do not wring it dry. The cloth should be moist with oil.

3 Position the cloth over the area you are going to treat.

4 Cover the cloth with plastic wrap or sheeting (plastic wrap can be wound around the body to secure the pack in place).

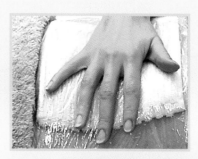

5 Then place a towel over the top of the plastic, and a hot-water bottle or hot pack over the towel.

6 Lie down for 30 to 40 minutes. Shower off when you are finished.

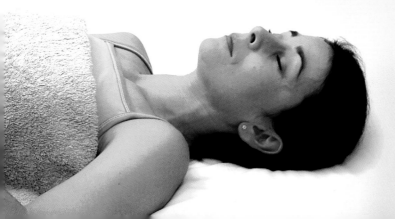

Dry Skin Brushing

Your body eliminates waste products through your skin. To maximize its effectiveness, your skin must be allowed to perform its eliminative function unimpaired. Restrictive artificial fabrics and antiperspirants negatively affect your skin's ability to do so. As well as avoiding these things, we also can stimulate the skin to work more effectively by employing a few simple techniques, including dry skin brushing. This exfoliates the skin and also stimulates the lymph and blood. It leaves you with a pleasant tingling glow, and over time your skin will attain a satin-like, youthful appearance.

CONDITIONS TO TREAT

Dry skin brushing can be used where there is a scurf rim, regardless of whether or not there is a skin problem. It is an aid to elimination, reduces the stress on the kidneys and is part of a general detox program. It improves skin condition, returning lack-luster skin to glowing positive health. You can perform skin brushing where there is a skin inflammation, as long as you don't brush over broken or weeping skin.

CONTRAINDICATIONS

Do not brush broken skin, acne, or weeping skin conditions such as eczema. Brush around raised moles.

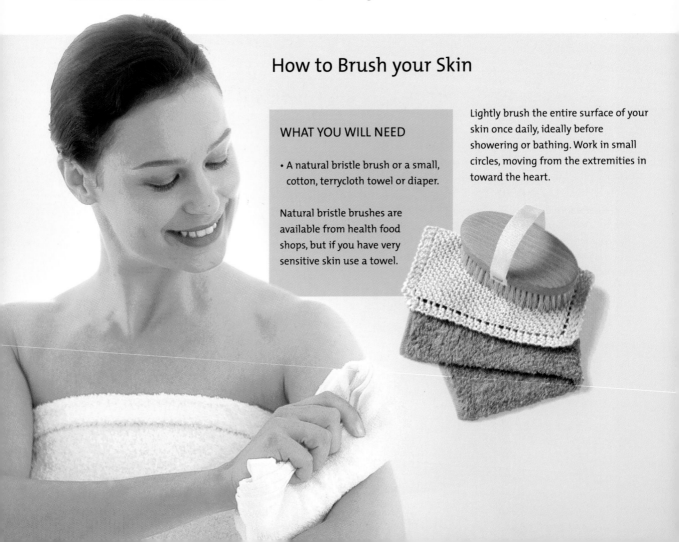

How to Brush your Skin

WHAT YOU WILL NEED

• A natural bristle brush or a small, cotton, terrycloth towel or diaper.

Natural bristle brushes are available from health food shops, but if you have very sensitive skin use a towel.

Lightly brush the entire surface of your skin once daily, ideally before showering or bathing. Work in small circles, moving from the extremities in toward the heart.

Water Consumption

Your body is composed of 70% water, and this needs constant cleaning and replacement. You need to drink an average of two liters of pure water a day, but if you drink alcohol, coffee, tea, or carbonated, sugary drinks, you need extra water to compensate for their dehydrating effects. Excess salt in your diet will also increase this need.

If you currently do not drink enough water, try to increase your daily intake over a period of a few weeks by setting yourself targets and increasing slowly. Once you have the habit of drinking more, you will find it easy to maintain, and you will notice the shortfall if you slacken off.

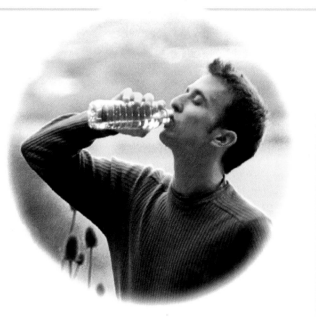

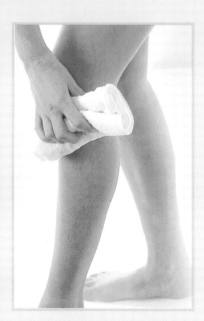

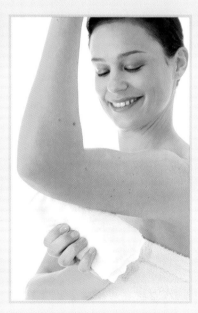

3 When you reach your abdomen, brush wide circles around your navel in a clockwise motion, about five times.

4 Finish by softly brushing your face. Start with your forehead, then work to each side and down past your ears. Brush outward over your cheekbones and down the side of your neck. Do the same over your upper lip and chin, working from the center out, and then down your neck. Finish by brushing down your neck, following the flow of lymphatic drainage.

Doing your back
If you like, use a long-handled natural-bristle brush to reach your back. Brush downward from the shoulders as far as you can reach.

1 Begin with your feet and work up your legs and over your buttocks.

2 Then brush your arms, beginning with your hands and working up to

your shoulders. Then brush around your rib cage in toward the center and around each breast.

Hydrotherapy

Water can be used to stimulate circulation and boost your skin's eliminative function, as well as that of the deeper organs of your body. It is a powerful adjunct to any health-building program.

Use hydrotherapy on a daily basis for best results. You can direct water at certain organs or parts of the body that need attention, for example, an aching joint or a congested liver or kidney. Simply by stimulating the circulation in these areas you will effectively mobilize your body's healing energy in that direction. Saunas and steam baths, with accompanying cold plunges, are included in hydrotherapy. Some spas have hoses that can be used to deliver high-pressure jets of water at specific locations on the body.

CONDITIONS TO TREAT

Hydrotherapy may be used as an integral part of a general detoxification program. However, it may be very successful in the treatment of all kinds of localized problems, from liver congestion to arthritis. It is particularly helpful in cases of chronic inflammation. Arthritic joints benefit not only from the increase in circulation, but also in a reduction in local pain. Water may be directed at specific sites, including the liver and kidneys, and other internal organs, in order to improve the circulation in those areas.

CONTRAINDICATIONS

Hypermobile joints should not be overheated and rheumatic joints should not be overchilled. Use warm/cool water if these problems apply. These conditions will improve over time, and tolerance will develop if you persevere.

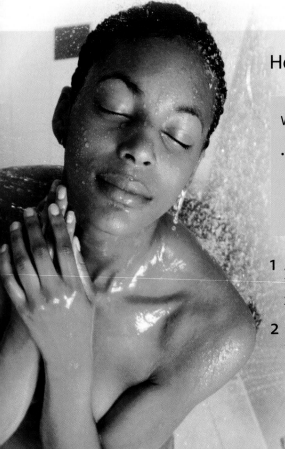

How to Perform Hydrotherapy

WHAT YOU WILL NEED

- A shower (or a bath with a shower attachment) with hot and cold water.

1 After you have performed dry skin brushing (see page 110), get into your shower or bath.

2 Direct water, as hot as you can stand for between 30 seconds to 1 minute, all over your body.

3 Then, with the water as cold as you can take for between 30 seconds to 1 minute, direct this over your body.

4 Perform this several times, each session lasting between 30 seconds to 1 minute. If you start with moderate temperatures, you will find that you can quickly progress to greater extremes of hot and cold.

5 Finish by using cold water if you can, though if you suffer from rheumatic or arthritic conditions, it is best to end by using warm water.

Bowel Cleanses

No detox is complete without attention to the bowel, the body's main exit channel. Cleansing the bowel with herbal remedies, enemas, or colonic hydrotherapy, can be an essential part of a healing program. Seek expert advice before performing these routines.

The rationale for bowel cleansing is that the health of the bowel is fundamental to the health of your whole system. Toxins retained in the bowel can leak into the surrounding tissues and the blood, affecting other organs, and may be at the root of many symptoms, such as tiredness, headaches, circulatory difficulties, menstrual and hormonal problems, and immune dysfunction.

Your first step to ensuring good bowel health is adequate hydration. Adults need to drink an average of 2 liters of water a day. It is vital that you drink adequate amounts of water if you undertake a bowel cleanse. One of the functions of the colon is to absorb water from the feces. If there is too little water, the feces become dry and sticky, making it more difficult for the body to get rid of them.

It should take about 10 to 12 hours for material to make the journey through your body. At least one bowel movement for each meal is ideal.

Herbal bowel cleanses operate on a dual principle of cathartic herbs, which stimulate the peristaltic muscles to evacuate, and mucilaginous and demulcent herbs, which soothe the lining of the bowel and provide bulk. Additionally, we add ingredients that absorb any matter stuck on the bowel wall, or in little pockets (diverticuloses) that most of us develop as we grow older.

CONDITIONS TO TREAT
Congestion, systemic toxicity, constipation, liver congestion, menstrual problems, headaches and throat and sinus problems.

CONTRAINDICATIONS
Consult a professional health practitioner if you have a serious medical condition. The full bowel cleanse may be contraindicated if you have an inflammatory bowel condition such as ulcerative colitis.

ESSENTIAL INGREDIENTS
Seek expert advice on how to perform a bowel cleanse. You can prepare bowel-moving capsules or a formula for absorbing impurities. For bowel-moving capsules, you will need:
- Powders of aloe, cascara, senna, ginger, cayenne, garlic, and barberry root bark. These stimulate peristalsis, correct the gastrointestinal environment, control candida, and boost the body's immunity.
For the formula to absorb impurities, you will need:
- Powders of psyllium husk, linseeds, fennel seeds, slippery elm inner bark, marshmallow root, activated charcoal, bentonite or French green clay, and apple pectin. This absorbs toxic matter, for elimination.

Enemas

These may be both curative, part of a "get well" program, or preventive. When performed on a regular basis they can strengthen and cleanse the body, increasing its resistance and general stamina. However, they should not be a replacement for natural bowel movements. If you are unable to establish a natural frequency of bowel motions, you should seek help from a herbalist or a colonic therapist.

Enema kits can be obtained for home use; however, it is very important that you get some advice, training, and guidance in how to use them from a trained practitioner.

The Kidney Flush or "Master Cleanser"

This tried and trusted naturopathic routine is simple and effective for detoxifying the kidneys. You can make this a regular morning routine, or use it on those mornings when you need extra help cleansing and detoxifying your body, for example, if you are feeling sluggish. Mornings are also times when your body is cleansing itself naturally. You will find this routine bracing and stimulating. Do not eat anything before drinking the kidney flush.

CONDITIONS TO TREAT

General congestion, sinusitis, water retention, mild arthritis or rheumatism, poor circulation.

CONTRAINDICATIONS

If you frequently experience excessive stomach acid and reflux, lemons may exacerbate this. In this case, use half a lemon only, or use apple cider vinegar instead.

How to Prepare the Kidney Flush

WHAT YOU WILL NEED

- Two lemons or one lemon and one lime, preferably organic and unwaxed
- A juicer
- Half a pint of pure water, cold or hot
- Cayenne tincture or cayenne powder
- Maple syrup to sweeten, if desired

1 Put the whole lemons and lime through the juicer. The skin and pith of citrus fruits contain many beneficial essential oils. Some people experience an occasional tendency to an over-acid stomach with these fruits, and the skin and pith counteract this.

2 Add the juice to at least half a pint of pure water. You can use either cold or hot water.

3 Add 10 drops of tincture of cayenne pepper, or a pinch of cayenne powder. If you need to sweeten the drink, add organic maple syrup, not sugar or honey.

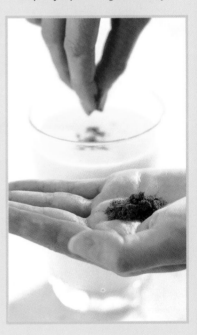

4 Do not eat anything until half an hour after finishing the flush.

The Liver Flush

This morning routine detoxifies the liver, stimulating it to cleanse itself by dumping bile through the biliary tract into the gastrointestinal tract, making you feel lighter and more energetic. It also is nourishing and supporting to both your immune system and digestion, and will help your body to throw off the threat of viral or bacterial infection.

Perform this routine first thing in the morning before eating. You may feel a little faint or sick at first, or develop a slight headache—this is temporary hypoglycemia (low blood sugar) as a result of not eating when you are used to. If you

persevere this will be cured by the routine. The garlic in the flush is a wonderful remedy for the pancreas, as it works to correct blood sugar imbalances and stimulates the secretion of digestive enzymes.

You should perform the kidney flush for a few days before you start on the liver flush. Then perform the liver flush for five days in a row, break for two days, then perform another five. You can repeat this flush any time you are feeling a bit sluggish, after overindulgence of any kind, or routinely at the change of the seasons, which is a time that tends to put stress on our systems.

CONDITIONS TO TREAT

General congestion, digestive bloating and fullness, low immunity, menstrual problems, allergies, persistent headaches (check with a medical practitioner first for more serious possibilities).

CONTRAINDICATIONS

If you have gallstones or a liver disease such as hepatitis, do not use this procedure without consulting a professional practitioner. If you are pregnant you may do this flush, however, substitute a simple herbal tea instead of the detox tea—peppermint is ideal.

How to Prepare the Liver Flush

WHAT YOU WILL NEED

- 1 lemon
- ½ pint organic fresh pressed apple juice
- 1 tablespoon virgin cold-pressed olive oil
- 1 clove garlic
- small piece fresh ginger root
- herbal detox tea (page 117)

- Do not eat anything before drinking the liver flush.

- Juice the lemon in a juicer.

- Crush then finely chop the garlic.

- Grate the ginger.

- Place all of the ingredients in a blender and liquidize.

- Pour out and drink slowly.

- Start preparing the herbal detox tea.

- Fifteen minutes after you have finished drinking the liver flush, sip at least two mugs of the detox tea slowly for the next hour or so. Do not eat anything for two hours after you start this routine, then preferably eat something light; fruit is ideal.

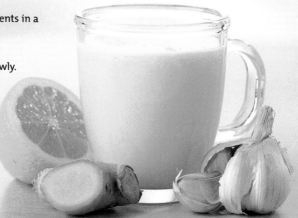

Herbal Preparations

Infusions, decoctions, tinctures, and teas have a wide range of applications. The preparation methods are the same, no matter your iris type, and each has been designed to make the most of the different parts of plants.

CONDITIONS TO TREAT

Throughout the book, you'll be recommended different herbal preparations for each constitution and problem. The herbal detox tea is used in conjunction with the liver flush (see page 115). You also can use it for general congestion, water retention, low immunity, and bloating.

CONTRAINDICATIONS

Specific recommendations are given for each drink, but avoid the detox tea if you are pregnant and, if you suffer from high blood pressure, omit the licorice.

Decoction

Use this method for roots, seeds, barks, and berries.

1 Place 1 dessertspoonful of dried herbs in a saucepan.

2 Add 1 pint of water, bring to a boil, and simmer for 10–15 minutes.

3 Strain and drink.

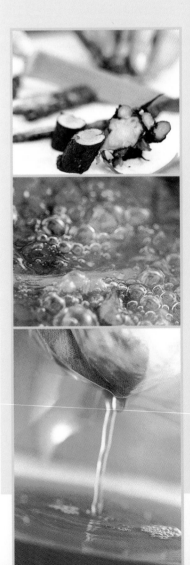

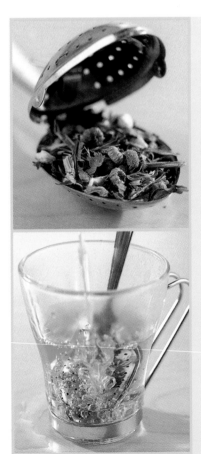

Infusion

Use this method for dried leaves, flowers, and "tops" of herbs.

1 Place 1 teaspoon of dried herbs in a tea infuser (a tisanniere or tea-ball).

2 Place the infuser in a cup. Pour freshly boiled water over the infuser.

3 Steep for 10 minutes and then drink the tea.

Alternatively, add 1 dessertspoonful of dried herbs to 1 pint of boiled water in a teapot. Steep, as above, and then drink.

Tinctures or Fluid Extracts

These are alcohol and water extractions, and are very concentrated. They are available from the larger herbal stores and health food shops, and from herbal practitioners. The dose depends on the strength of the extract, but a rough guide is one teaspoon three times a day for tinctures, or half a teaspoon three times a day for fluid extracts.

Herbal Detox Tea

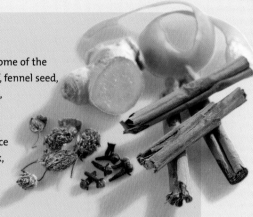

WHAT YOU WILL NEED

- 1 heaped dessertspoon of all or some of the following herbs: peppermint leaf, fennel seed, fresh ginger rhizome, nettle herb, yellow dock root, dandelion root, burdock root, red clover flowers, fenugreek seed, clove buds, licorice root, orange peel, Pau d'Arco bark, juniper berry, black peppercorn, cinnamon bark, cardamom pods
- 2 pints water

1 Either steep the herbs for 15 minutes in hot water, or, for a stronger effect, place 1 heaped dessertspoonful in a pan.

2 Add 1 pint of water, bring to the boil, and simmer for 10 minutes.

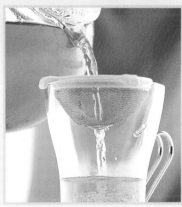

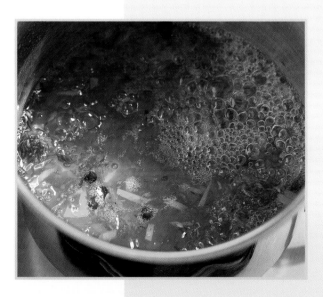

3 Strain the herbs, replace them in the pan with another pint of water, and then repeat.

Do not drink this tea if you are pregnant, and if you have high blood pressure, omit the licorice.

Deep Breathing

As well as helping you feel generally centered and energized, deep breathing is very effective for keeping lymph active. The main lymphatic vessel is the thoracic duct, which passes directly through the diaphragm. As the diaphragm moves with your breath, the thoracic duct is massaged, drawing lymph through your entire system. Most of us breathe shallowly, from our chests, which, apart from preventing us from receiving adequate oxygenation, does not engage the diaphragm.

Deep breathing can be integrated into the busiest lifestyle with some discipline and application. The most important thing is to be comfortable. It can be performed while sitting, lying, or standing. If you are standing, make sure you are standing straight, with your feet hip-width apart; your knees loose, not locked; and your arms relaxed by your sides.

VISUALIZATION

If you wish, as you breathe in, imagine your body filling with white or golden light, penetrating to the deepest parts of yourself. As you breathe out, visualize all the tension, blockages, negativity, toxicity, and congestion flowing out of you.

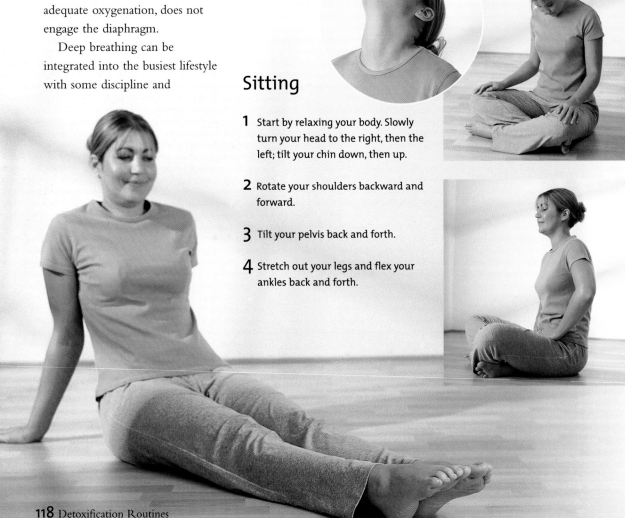

Sitting

1 Start by relaxing your body. Slowly turn your head to the right, then the left; tilt your chin down, then up.

2 Rotate your shoulders backward and forward.

3 Tilt your pelvis back and forth.

4 Stretch out your legs and flex your ankles back and forth.

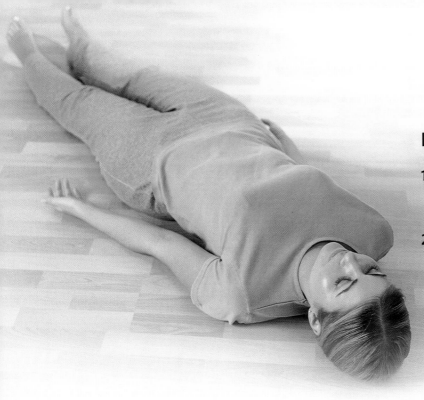

Lying Down

1 Ensure that your body is aligned symmetrically. Perform a brief check on your limbs and muscles.

2 Starting with your feet and moving upward, relax each part of your body in turn. When you get to your head, also pay attention to your eyes and throat, making sure to consciously release any tension you find in these areas.

Performing Deep Breathing

1 Begin to breathe in slowly and evenly, drawing your breath deep into your abdomen. Place your hands over your abdomen so that you can feel it rise with your in-breath.

2 Keep breathing in until your breath reaches your upper chest. Do not hold your breath.

3 Release your breath by letting it go naturally, letting gravity take it out with no effort on your part.

4 Repeat this pattern at least ten times on each occasion, and perform the routine as often as you find it helpful. Upon completing the cycle you should feel energized, restored, and enlivened.

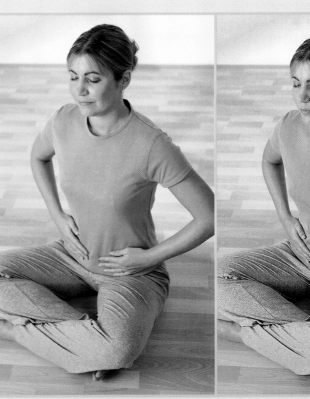
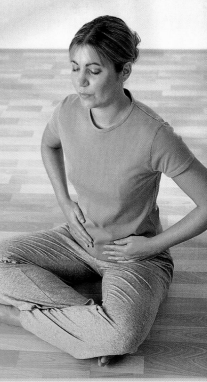

Stretching

The following exercises allow your body to release tension and also occupy your mind. They can specifically help high resistance types (see pages 40–43) reduce caffeine and sugar in their diet, if performed habitually at the onset of any cravings they may experience.

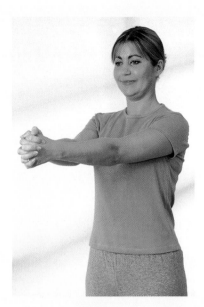

How to Perform Stretching Exercises

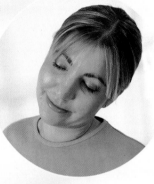

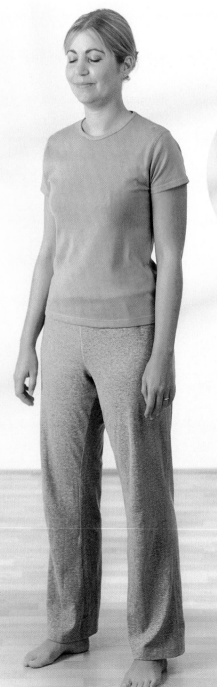

1 Stand up. Start by stretching your neck and head, rolling your head from side to side.

2 Bring your shoulders as far up toward your ears as you can, then drop them. Do this several times, then roll your shoulders forward and backward a few times.

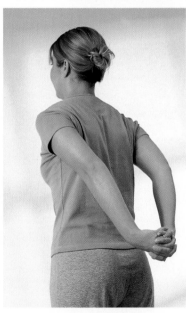

3 Clasp your hands in front of you and pull them forward, feeling the stretch across your upper back. Then clasp your hands behind you and pull gently backward, feeling the stretch in your upper chest.

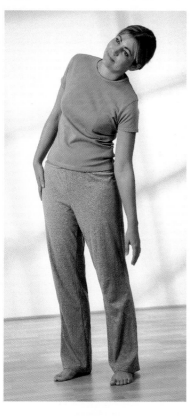

4 Next, bend first to one side, letting your fingers slide down the outside of your thighs as far as you can comfortably go, then the other.

5 Circle your hips a few times, first one way, then the other.

6 Stretch one leg out in front of you, bend your other leg, and bend forward over the stretched leg, feeling the pull on the back of your thigh and calf. Repeat on the other side.

7 Finally, let yourself hang forward, with your knees soft and your arms and hands hanging loose toward your feet. Breathe deeply and relax for a few seconds. When you have finished, be sure to drink a full tumbler of water.

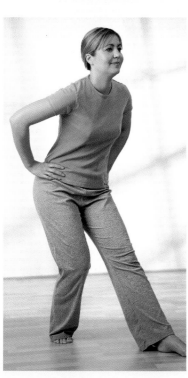

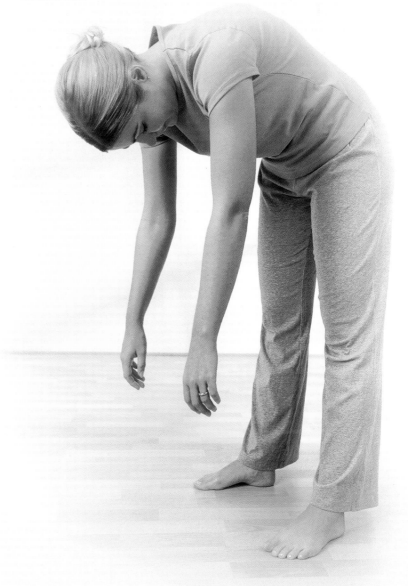

Visualization

Visualization is used chiefly to reinforce positive messages and improve self-esteem. It also aids meditation, rest, and relaxation.

How to Perform a Visualization

1 Sit, lie down, or stand—whatever is most comfortable for you. Close your eyes and imagine you are in a beautiful location of your choice. This may be somewhere real already known to you, or it may be an imagined location. Make sure to see the detail of the place—what is the landscape like, what colors and textures do you see, what sounds do you hear, what smells do you notice?

2 Make yourself as comfortable as you can in this location. Imagine that everything you could possibly need is readily available to you, that whatever you desire can be manifested immediately. Play with this thought a little, without guilt or judgment. You may fantasize about a delicious meal, for example.

3 When you have satisfied this desire, imagine that you are now free to travel through your own world and create whatever you want in your life. Think of the various different aspects of your life—job, money, relationship, leisure, etc., and imagine how they would be if they were perfect. Go into detail and allow yourself to fantasize absolute perfection. Brush aside any cynical thoughts that come into your mind telling you that you can never attain this perfection.

4 If there is a particularly difficult problem you are faced with, imagine that it is completely and effortlessly resolved. It doesn't matter what it is—it may be giving up smoking or finding a new job. Whatever it is, focus on the successful end result, not the problems of achieving it. Imagine that you have already achieved it.

5 When you have this feeling of success, return again to your ideal location. Look around and take in the environment, before bidding it goodbye, till your next visit, then slowly return to the outside world.

6 Always visualize absolute perfection, and do not analyze your fantasy. Simply regard it as a positive seed that you have planted, which you are sure will grow into fruition in good time. Wait with certainty and optimism for it to manifest.

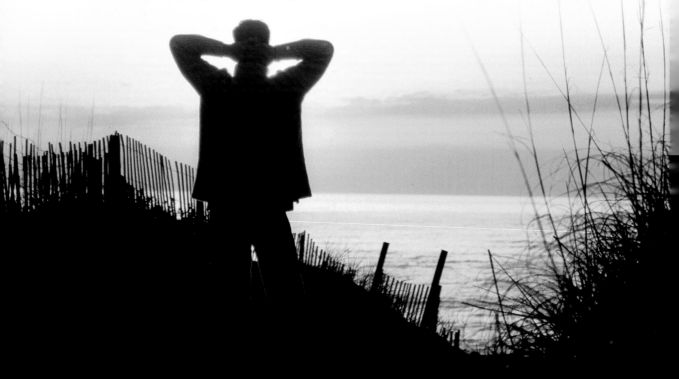

Food Combining

Eating and drinking foods in particular combinations can be invaluable for weight loss and for treating certain digestive disorders, as one of its benefits is to facilitate the eliminative functions and maximize digestive power. Well-known versions include the Hay diet, and the "Fit for Life" program.

CONDITIONS TO TREAT

Obesity and weight problems, blood sugar abnormalities, digestive bloating, acid indigestion, and food allergies/sensitivities.

CONTRAINDICATIONS

None.

HOW TO PERFORM FOOD-COMBINING

- Eat fruit only for breakfast. You can eat as much as you like, but try not to eat too many different types at one sitting. In particular, do not combine melons with other fruits. Melon is digested very easily and quickly, even more so than other fruits. If combined with other foods it tends to ferment, causing bloating and discomfort. You may, however, take one of the "superfood" formulae available, see box, right. Your first full meal should be at lunchtime.

- Never eat fruit with any other food type, so don't have it for dessert after a main meal. You need to leave at least half an hour between eating fruit and anything else, and at least two hours after eating a meal before you eat fruit.

- Do not drink anything with your meals except a moderate quantity of water, a herbal digestive tea, or vegetable juice. Drinking anything else will dilute digestive secretions and weaken your digestion.

- If you eat animal proteins, separate these from any carbohydrates. Alternating between proteins and carbohydrates on a day-to-day basis can work well. This probably will require a fairly radical reworking of your diet as the protein/carbohydrate combination is at the heart of many popular dishes. However, the pancreas, particularly, is eased considerably by not having to work so hard, and you end up having much better digestion.

- Never eat after 8 pm. At this time your digestive powers are virtually dormant. Food eaten after this will lie heavily on your stomach, and may not in fact move far until morning, perhaps contributing to restless and disturbed sleep patterns.

Superfoods

This is the name given to natural vegetable and plant foods containing above average nutrition. They may be single foods—alfalfa and other sprouted seeds; spirulina, chlorella, and blue/green algae—all of which are fresh water algae, and sea vegetables. The latter are particularly rich in minerals. There also are proprietary brands available, combining several sources in one formula, usually in powder form.

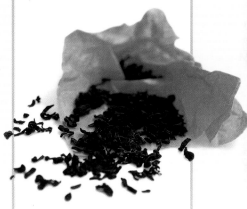

CONDITIONS TO TREAT
Fatigue/low energy, immune deficiency, and digestive difficulties (superfoods supply easy energy in cases where digestion struggles to do so). Superfoods also combat the effects of stress and supply extra quantities of nutrients—vitamins, minerals, trace elements, and micronutrients.

CONTRAINDICATIONS
Check the ingredients for substances to which you may be allergic, otherwise there are no contraindications.

A Glossary of Iridology Terms

[NB: terms in bold type refer to items that may be looked up elsewhere in the glossary.]

ABSORPTION RING (pupillary ruff) Describes the narrow ring of pigmented tissue at the inner pupil border (**IPB**); called the absorption ring as it is said by some researchers (notably Jensen) to depict the functionality (i.e. absorption capacity) of the inner surface of the gastrointestinal tract.

ACUTE An active process having generally a short and relatively severe effect (e.g. fever, inflammation). Opposite of **chronic**.

ANTERIOR BORDER LAYER The surface layer of the iris, in which **pathochromic signs** may appear, due to the presence of pigment cells that are contained in this layer. The ABL is then also encased in a thin endothelial membrane.

ANTERIOR CHAMBER The fluid-filled space behind the **cornea**, in front of the **iris**.

ANW The Autonomic Nerve Wreathe, also known as **Collarette**, the concentric vascular structure which divides the iris disk in two parts, roughly a third of the way into the **stroma** from the **pupillary margin**.

ARCUS SENILIS Also called the "arcus," consists of a partial ring of whitish plaque in the **cornea**, generally obscuring the outer zone of the iris frontally (sometimes also ventrally), considered to be a deposition of cholesterol, triglycerides, inorganic sodium, and other detritus that may block the arteries. "Senilis" suggests this is usually seen in older people. *See also* **lipemic annulus**.

CENTRAL HETEROCHROMIA Pigment located over the central portion of the iris only, covering the **pupillary zone**, and also perhaps the **collarette** and **humoral zone**. Signifies potential for disturbances of the GI tract.

CERVICAL Pertaining to the neck.

CHRONIC Long-term pathology, may involve degeneration and nerve damage.

Associated with dark signs in the iris. Opposite of **acute**.

CILIARY ZONE The outer two thirds (approximately) of the iris disk, between the **collarette** and the **limbus**.

COLLARETTE The concentric vascular structure that divides the iris into two parts, roughly two thirds of the way into the stroma from the **pupillary margin**. *See also* ANW.

CONSTITUTION The makeup and functional habit of the body as determined by the genetic endowment of the individual, and modified by environmental and lifestyle factors.

CONTRACTION FURROWS Circular grooves or furrows in the anterior layers of the iris. Several may appear at once in a concentric pattern. They may circle the iris disk entirely or only partially, and may also be broken in places. They signal the effects of stress upon the system, neuromuscular holding patterns, mineral deficiencies, and metabolic imbalances mediated through the nervous system. Also termed **nerve rings** and **cramp rings**.

CORNEA The transparent membrane that protects the anterior aspect of the eye, partly encapsulating the **anterior chamber**.

CRAMP RING *see* **contraction furrow**.

CRYPT A small dark opening, often rhomboid in shape, in the texture of the iris **stroma**. Almost invariably found at or near, either inside or outside, the collarette.

DEFECT SIGN Also known as "defect of substance": a small, black mark, often found inside a **crypt** or **lacuna**. Signifies degenerative process.

DENSITY A measure of the proximity of iris fibers to each other. Determines **resistance** and recuperative powers.

DEPIGMENTATION Loss of pigment or color in the iris. It has been assumed in some iridology circles that this is a sign of reestablishment of health: however, in some

cases depigmentation may be pathological, i.e. caused by disease, viral, or autoimmune disturbance.

DIATHESIS Higher than average tendency to acquire certain pathologies; regulatory dysfunction which may be either inherited or acquired.

DISPOSITION Term referring to **density** and structure of the iris (Hauser), depicting inherent level and distribution of vitality, **resistance**, and the consequent likely behavior of the individual **constitution**.

DYSCHROMIA *see* **pathochromic sign** assumption of metabolic disturbance signified by pigments in the iris.

EPITHELIUM The exterior or interior (sometimes called "endothelium") lining of any organ.

FLOCCULATIONS Light-colored flaky masses usually appearing in the outer zone of the iris.

HETEROCHROMIA Hetero = different; chromia = color.

HONEYCOMB A **lacuna** with several "chambers."

HUMORAL ZONE The zone immediately outside the **collarette**. Describes the deep cardiovascular and lymphatic circulation, and has implications for absorption and distribution of nutrients; also hormonal activity.

HYPER Increased.

HYPO Decreased, diminished.

IPB The inner pupil border: the inner edge of the iris.

LACUNA An opening in the iris **stroma**, usually appearing as an oval hole in the texture, although other shapes are frequently seen. Lacunae may be "closed," (completely surrounded or bordered by a fiber structure), or "open," (only partially surrounded or bordered).

LEAF LACUNA A lacuna found just outside the **collarette**, with fibers inside resembling the ribs of a leaf. Signifies functional disturbance of the hollow and hormonal organs.

LESION A break or breakdown of tissue or texture. In iridology terms a lesion is usually synonymous with a **lacuna** or **crypt**.

LIMBUS The meeting of the outer edge of the iris and the **sclera**.

LIPEMIC ANNULUS Opaque whitish ring circling the entire outer zone of the iris; also known (incorrectly) as a cholesterol ring. To be distinguished from the **arcus senilis**.

LYMPHATIC ROSARY A ring of **tophi** or **flocculations** in the outer iris zone (usually fifth minor), found in the hydrogenoid constitution, signifying tendency towards lymphatic stasis.

MEDUSA A type of lacuna usually found in the lung or kidney **reaction fields**, resembling the head of snakes of the mythical monster. Also known as a "jellyfish lacuna."

NASAL Term of orientation: that side of the iris close to the nose.

NERVE RINGS see **contraction furrows**.

NUTRITIVE ZONE also known as the **pupillary zone**, so called as it contains the **reaction field** for the gastrointestinal tract.

PATHOCHROMIC SIGN A pigment marking in the **anterior border layer** of the iris. To be distinguished from **sectoral/central heterochromia**. May appear in a variety of colors from pale yellow to dark brown, color indicating the focus of potential pathology.

POSTERIOR Situated toward the rear.

POSTERIOR EPITHELIUM A darkly pigmented iris layer that serves to prevent the penetration of light through the iris into the posterior chamber of the eye.

POSTERIOR MEMBRANE The dilator layer of the iris consisting of a thin layer of plain muscle fiber.

PUPILLARY MARGIN Inner edge of the iris bordering the pupil. *See also* **IPB**.

PUPILLARY RUFF The structure at the inner margin of the pupil, appearing as a red/orange "ruff": it consists of the outermost portion of the **retina** as it curls under the **IPB**. It is an extension of the optic nerve and is the only portion of the nervous system visible to the eye.

PUPILLARY ZONE Section of the iris bordered by the **collarette** and the IPB. Also known as the **nutritive zone**.

RADIAL FURROW A radiating crease in the iris tissue, wide at the base and tapered toward the limbus. Major radials start in the **pupillary zone** and cross the **collarette**; minor radials start at the collarette and proceed toward the limbus.

RADII SOLARIS Another name for **radial furrows**.

RAREFACTION A focal loosening in the fiber structure of the iris **stroma**, indicating lack of resistance in the relevant **reaction field**.

REACTION FIELD Topographical sector of the iris where information is registered.

REACTIVITY The ability of the organism to react to threats from toxicity or pathogens: shown by relative shading of the iris stroma or trabeculae.

RESISTANCE Ability of the organism to resist morbid or threatening influences. Shown by the relative **density** of iris **stroma**.

RETINA The innermost tunic of the eye, an expansion or continuation of the optic nerve, forming the receptor for visual sensation.

ROOT TRANSVERSAL A **transversal** with two or more branches.

SCHNABEL LACUNA *Schnabel* means "beak": sometimes called a "beak lacuna." A lacuna with a sharp point penetrating the **collarette**, signifying a potential tumor. The point of the beak may be rounded (benign) or straight (malignant).

SCLERA The white of the eye: an opaque fibrous membrane which protects the inner eye from injury.

SCURF RIM A darkened outer zone indicating a reflux or reabsorption of toxic material from a poorly eliminating skin.

SECTORAL HETEROCHROMIA Pigmentation of a distinct radial sector of the iris.

SPHINCTER PUPILLAE A muscular band in the **nutritive/pupillary zone** of the iris, which contracts the pupil.

SPONDAL-ARTHRITIC RING White frosting at the border between the sclera and the iris, usually **nasal**, occasionally **temporal**. Predisposition to arthritis, calcium loss, osteoporosis.

STROMA The vascular layer constituting the bulk of the iris.

TEMPORAL Term of orientation: that portion of the iris closest to the temple.

TRABECULA (plural trabeculae) The vascular fibers that comprise the iris stroma.

TRANSVERSAL A trabecular fiber that runs "across the grain."

TOPHI *see* **flocculations**.

TOPOLABILE Name given to a sign that is significant for its general appearance, rather than its precise topographical position on the iris chart.

TOPOSTABILE Name given to a sign that is important for its precise topographical position on the iris chart.

VASCULARIZATION Loss of the outer sheath of an iris fiber (**trabecula**). The fiber then appears to have a pink thread running through it. A sign of stress or trauma to the organ in the relevant **reaction field**.

VENTRAL Term of orientation: the lower portion of the iris.

Index

Acknowledgments

The author would like to thank: Anji Jackson-Main for unending love, support and encouragement; Richard Schulze for expanding my concepts of health and disease beyond anything I had previously envisioned; Harri Wolf for his clear and precise teaching and for his inspired interpretations, which have fuelled many years of my own research; Michelle Bernard for the original encouragement to write this book; all at Carroll & Brown for making this work as pleasant as it has been to consummate; Angela and Peter Bradbury, Jill Davies, Farida Sharan, Harri Wolf and Ellen Tart-Jensen for their willing assistance; my mother and father, wife Anji and children Seth, Aaron, Jasper and Chloe for first-hand experience of the miracle of heredity, and for pressing the buttons that make sense of life; all the pioneers of iridology, who have been vital in some measure in the shaping of the material here presented.

Carroll & Brown would like to thank:
Production Director Karol Davies
Production Controller Nigel Reed
Computer Management Paul Stradling
Additional Design Assistance Jim Cheatle
Photographer Jules Selmes
Photographer's Assistant David Yems
Picture Researcher Sandra Schneider
Proofreader Geoffrey West
Indexer Michelle Bernard

Picture Credits

p12 and 13 (top) The Guild of Naturopathic Iridologists, 94 Grosvenor Road, London SW1 3LF Tel/fax 020 7821 0255 www.gni-international.orgp
p13 (bottom) David Christopher www.herballegacy.com
p108 (top) Brian Carter/Garden Picture Library
p108 (bottom) Imagesprite.com
p109 Imagesprite.com
p122 John Henley/Corbis

Useful Websites

holistic.iridology@ntlworld.com
www.thenaturalcentre.com
www.gni-international.org
www.associationofmasterherbalists.co.uk

Suggested Further Reading

Hall, Dorothy, *Iridology: How the Eyes Reveal Your Health and Personality*, Keats Publishing, 1981
Jensen, Bernard and Bodeen, Donald V, *Visions of Health*, Avery, 1992
Sharan, Farida, *Iridology: A Complete Guide to Diagnosing Through the Iris and to Related Forms of Treatment*, Thorsons, 1986
Sharan, Farida, *Herbs of Grace*, Wisdome Press, 1994
Johnson, Denny Ray *What the Eye Reveals*, Rayid Publications, 2nd edn, 1997
Dethefsen Thorwald and Dahlke, Rudiger *The Healing Power of Illness: The Meaning of Symptoms and How to Interpret Them*, Sterling, 2002